HEALTH CARE AND CHRISTIAN ETHICS

How can Christian ethics make a significant contribution to health care ethics in today's Western, pluralistic society? Robin Gill examines the 'moral gaps' in secular accounts of health care ethics and the tensions within specifically theological accounts. He explores the healing stories in the Synoptic Gospels, identifying four core virtues present within them – compassion, care, faith and humility – that might bring greater depth to a purely secular interpretation of health care ethics. Each of these virtues is examined in turn, using a range of topical issues including health care rationing, genetics, HIV/AIDS, withholding/withdrawing nutrition from PVS patients, and the empirical evidence which suggests a connection between religion and health. Professor Gill also argues that these four virtues are shared by other major religious and humanistic traditions and that, together with secular principles, they can enrich health care ethics even in a pluralistic society.

ROBIN GILL is Michael Ramsey Professor of Modern Theology at University of Kent, Canterbury. He is series editor of New Studies in Christian Ethics, author of *Churchgoing and Christian Ethics* (1999) and editor of *The Cambridge Companion to Christian Ethics* (2000). Professor Gill is Chair of the Archbishop of Canterbury's Medical Ethics Advisory Group and a member of the BMA Medical Ethics Committee, although he writes here in his own capacity.

NEW STUDIES IN CHRISTIAN ETHICS

General Editor: Robin Gill
Editorial Board: Stephen R. L. Clark, Stanley Hauerwas, Robin W. Lovin

Christian ethics has increasingly assumed a central place within academic theology. At the same time the growing power and ambiguity of modern science and the rising dissatisfaction within the social sciences about claims to value-neutrality have prompted renewed interest in ethics within the secular academic world. There is, therefore, a need for studies in Christian ethics which, as well as being concerned with the relevance of Christian ethics to the present day secular debate, are well informed about parallel discussions in recent philosophy, science or social science. *New Studies in Christian Ethics* aims to provide books that do this at the highest intellectual level and demonstrate that Christian ethics can make a distinctive contribution to this debate – either in moral substance or in terms of underlying moral justifications.

New Studies in Christian Ethics

Titles published in the series:

HEALTH CARE AND CHRISTIAN ETHICS

ROBIN GILL

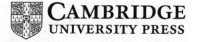

CAMBRIDGE
UNIVERSITY PRESS

CAMBRIDGE UNIVERSITY PRESS
Cambridge, New York, Melbourne, Madrid, Cape Town, Singapore, São Paulo

CAMBRIDGE UNIVERSITY PRESS
The Edinburgh Building, Cambridge CB2 2RU, UK

Published in the United States of America by Cambridge University Press, New York

www.cambridge.org
Information on this title: www.cambridge.org/9780521857239

First published 2006

Printed in the United Kingdom at the University Press, Cambridge

A catalogue record for this book is available from the British Library

ISBN-13 978-0-521-85723-9 hardback
ISBN-10 0-521-85723-6 hardback

Contents

Series editor's preface

This book is the twenty-sixth in the series New Studies in Christian Ethics, and the second contribution by its distinguished General Editor, Robin Gill. The author of *Health Care and Christian Ethics* ably advances the twin goals he has set for the series as a whole. The book both engages the secular moral debate about health care at the highest intellectual level and demonstrates the distinctive contribution of Christian ethics to that discussion. In so doing, Professor Gill illuminates many of the changes that have taken place in medical ethics and moral theory in recent decades.

At one point, medical ethics seemed a textbook example of the synthesis between Christian tradition and secular ethics. Christian ethicists initially took a leading role in framing principles of autonomy, physician responsibility, and patient rights for public use in health care settings. Application of the principles to specific questions of medical practice could then proceed independently of religious authority, but without hostility or indifference to religious traditions.

The terms of the discussion have changed dramatically, both in medicine and in ethics. Specialists in health care ethics now find the principles that shaped the discipline in its early days too abstract to be helpful apart from a rich cultural context that shapes use of principles and forms the character of those who offer care. This concern that moral principles, taken by themselves, are too 'thin' to offer real guidance converges with a broader development in moral philosophy which focuses on communities of virtue, rather than on autonomous agents making principled decisions about discrete moral questions.

However, this apparent agreement on the new shape of moral discourse quickly evaporates. Both philosophers and theologians often emphasise the importance of extended and highly developed traditions which can hardly be approximated in the pluralistic institutional settings of contemporary health care. The language of Christian theology, with its eschatological and Christological convictions, becomes for some the necessary precondition for meaningful moral discussion. On this view, public discussions in secular society simply lack the coherence necessary to provide real moral direction.

Robin Gill begins *Health Care and Christian Ethics* by setting the questions of health care ethics in the context of this larger debate about virtue ethics and the possibility of public theology. He then takes up the challenge of identifying values that are specifically grounded in Christian moral traditions about health and care, beginning with an extensive study of healing in the Synoptic Gospels. With a particularity that might have been disqualifying in the earlier search for general principles, he identifies four core values – compassion, care, faith and humility – that emerge from the Synoptic tradition and provide the basis for a critical Christian stance towards health and health care practices today.

Robin Gill's work has, however, also been characterised by realistic social assessments that refuse to take religious claims to moral uniqueness at face value. Alongside the distinctive values and virtues of the Christian heritage, he traces the interaction of Christian communities with other traditions and with the wider society. His earlier title in this series, *Churchgoing and Christian Ethics*, showed that the implementation of distinctive religious values is shaped by relationships with other aspects of the culture, even as the church contributes some version of its values to the wider discussion. Attentiveness to social reality should make us cautious supposing that theology alone guides the implementation of the core values of compassion, care, faith and humility or that persons outside of the tradition will find those values incomprehensible.

Robin Gill's study of Christian values in relation to the practical issues of health care recalls other titles in this series which have focused on specific problem areas, including Michael Northcott's *The Environment and Christian Ethics*, Peter Sedgwick's *The Market Economy and Christian Ethics*, and Douglas Hicks' study of urban society in *Inequality and Christian Ethics*. The exploration of specific Christian values connects with Garth Hallett's *Priorities and Christian Ethics*, and the study of the Synoptic healing stories returns to the issues raised in Ian McDonald's *Biblical Interpretation and Christian Ethics*. To think about health care in the terms Robin Gill provides leads us beyond those specific issues into a discussion of Christianity's contemporary public role that has also been presented in David Fergusson's *Community, Liberalism and Christian Ethics*, Robert Gascoigne's *The Public Forum and Christian Ethics* and David Hollenbach's *The Common Good and Christian Ethics*. Professor Gill's mastery of this broad range of literature and questions has given us an important book which contributes to health care ethics and illuminates new possibilities for the wider discussion about public theology.

ROBIN W. LOVIN

Acknowledgements

Many different people have helped to shape this book. However I am particularly grateful to Robin Lovin for his generous Preface, to Kate Brett and Kevin Taylor at Cambridge University Press for their expert editorial guidance over the years and to the anonymous reviewers they carefully selected. One of these was easy to unmask after so many years of friendship; Alastair Campbell, my former colleague at Edinburgh University and happily still a colleague on a number of national medical ethics committees, went the extra mile and commented helpfully on the whole text. In addition, my colleagues at the University of Kent have generously given their time reading parts of the text, especially John Court with his immense New Testament expertise, Alan Le Grys, Chris Cook (now at Durham) with his specialist medical expertise and my new colleagues Jeremy Carrette and Chris Deacy with their intelligence, friendship, enthusiasm and encouragement.

I am most grateful to colleagues at quite a number of conferences – including the national conference of hospital chaplains, the Society for the Study of Christian Ethics, the British Sociological Association's Sociology of Religion Study Group, British Medical Association's Study Conferences, and various parish-based conferences on medical ethics – as well as to numerous postgraduate students in medical ethics at the University of Kent. I have always found it immensely helpful to test out ideas on colleagues and students alike before committing them to print. Health care ethics can sometimes become too individualistic. The illustration reproduced on the cover of this book, from the glorious Edward Burne-Jones window at Birmingham Cathedral, depicts a more communal perspective, as well as pointing to the virtues of compassion, care, faith and humility that are so central to this study.

I gratefully acknowledge that a number of journals and edited books have allowed me to publish earlier versions of some of the ideas contained in this book: 'Autonomy in Medical Ethics After O'Neill' (with Gordon M. Stirrat), *Journal of Medical Ethics*, 31:2 (2005), pp. 127–30; 'Religious Membership', in William Schweiker (ed.), *The Blackwell Companion to Religious Ethics* (Oxford: Blackwell, 2005), pp. 493–500; 'Theological Purity versus Theological Realism', *Crucible*, 43:1 (January 2004), pp. 37–42; 'Public Theology and Genetics', in William F. Storrar and Andrew R. Morton (eds.), *Public Theology for the 21st Century* (Edinburgh: T. & T. Clark, 2004), pp. 253–66; 'Gospel Values and Modern Bioethics', in Martyn Percy and Stephen Lowe (eds.), *The Character of Wisdom: Essays in Honour of Wesley Carr* (Aldershot: Ashgate 2004), pp. 141–55; 'Health Care, Jesus and the Church', *Ecclesiology*, 1:1 (2004), pp. 37–55; 'Research Ethics (Human Participants) Committee: Working Principles' (with Richard Norman), University of Kent, www.kent.ac.uk, 26/8/2002; and 'Health Care and Covenant: Withholding and Withdrawing Treatment', in Mark J. Cartledge and David Mills (eds.), *Covenant Theology: Contemporary Approaches* (Carlisle and Waynesboro, GA: Paternoster Press, 2001), pp. 101–16.

Finally Jenny has been my loving companion for forty years. In moments of medical confusion while writing this book it has been especially good to have a doctor in the house.

Introduction

This book is written for all those who are interested in exploring whether and how Christian ethics might be able to make a significant contribution to health care ethics today in the public forum of a Western, pluralistic society.

A generation ago such exploration might have been considered largely unnecessary. Many of the pioneers of modern health care ethics were hospital chaplains, church leaders or academic theologians. In the 1960s the American theologian Paul Ramsey, and later William F. May, anticipated many of the issues that have now become commonplace in health care ethics. In Britain Bob Lambourne and his successors at Birmingham, followed by Gordon Dunstan at London, were instrumental in nurturing an interest in ethical and pastoral issues in medicine. In addition, a number of experienced hospital chaplains, such as Norman Autton at St George's Hospital, London, and church leaders, such as John Habgood and Ted Shotter, were also key pioneers.

Yet within a generation the discipline – variously termed health care ethics, medical ethics, biomedical ethics, bioethics, or ethics in medicine[1] – has become largely secularised. An important factor here is that secular philosophers and academic lawyers – such as Ian Kennedy in London, John Harris in Manchester, Sheila McLean in Glasgow and Peter Singer, first in Australia and now in the United States – are now leading voices in health care ethics. They offer distinctive legal and philosophical skills that bring new clarity to the developing discipline. In addition, it is often maintained that they

[1] I prefer the term health care ethics here because it includes ethics involved in both healing and health care provision (in medical, as well as genetic, science).

bring a more 'neutral' basis to health care ethics within a society increasingly perceived to be pluralistic and multi-cultural. Pluralism, multi-culturalism and what is often termed 'globalisation',[2] have particularly impacted upon health care in the Western world. It is just about plausible to argue that some sections of the population even in the West effectively live in enclaves and are little affected by globalisation. Yet in health care there are factors that make this less likely: overseas doctors and nurses are now extensively recruited from both northern and southern hemispheres; there is considerable travel to international medical conferences; and there are frequent reports in the international media and internet on novel health care issues. Within this specific context, it has become less acceptable to identify Britain, let alone the whole of the West, as 'Christian', so, it is often argued, health care ethics needs to be moulded in an explicitly secular direction. However well intentioned the work of the pioneer ethicists from the churches, the discipline clearly ought to be relevant to doctors, nurses and patients whatever their country of origin, religion, culture or ideological commitments. More than that, in areas of sharp controversy involving medical practice (despite frequent protestations from English Law Lords that they are not experts in medical ethics) the judicial system has increasingly become the final arbiter. In a pluralistic society judges rather than bishops – and lawyers rather than theologians – may now be considered to be the most appropriate arbiters.

This pattern of secularisation can be viewed in quite different ways within Christian ethics. On one understanding of secularisation[3] it is yet another example of the marginalisation of religion in modern society. It is part of a larger process involving the gradual erosion of religious beliefs, practices and institutions in the Western

---

[2] For a recent summary of the connection between pluralism and globalisation in the context of Christian ethics, see William Schweiker, *Theological Ethics and Global Dynamics: In the Time of Many Worlds* (New York and London: Blackwell, 2004).

[3] See the following collections for a variety of understandings of secularisation and modernity: Philip E. Hammond (ed.), *The Sacred in a Secular Age* (Berkeley: University of California Press, 1984); James A. Beckford and Thomas Luckmann (eds.), *The Changing Face of Religion* (London: Sage, 1989); Steve Bruce (ed.), *Religion and Modernization* (Oxford: Oxford University Press, 1992); and Alasdair Crocket and Richard O'Leary (eds.), *Patterns and Processes of Religious Change in Modern Industrial Societies – Europe and the United States* (Lampeter: Mellen, 2004).

world. Temporarily theologians and church leaders in the 1960s thought that they had discovered an area – namely health care ethics – in which they could uniquely contribute even within a largely secular society. Yet secular ethicists have now appropriated even this area for themselves. Moreover, this secular appropriation has taken place both in Britain/Europe and in the United States. There is no so-called European exceptionalism apparent here. Secular philosophy and academic law, and not theology, now dominate public health care ethics throughout the Western world, even in the United States (despite continuing high levels of private religious commitment there).

A quite different understanding of secularisation argues that it is the social function of churches to mould society at large in a more Christian direction. Once a particular change has been reliably initiated, churches can then return to their central function of worship and prayer. Just as there were a number of Christians who were instrumental in establishing the welfare state and the national health service in Britain in the 1940s, so there were also Christians who pioneered health care ethics in the 1960s. But, once their work was achieved, it was crucial that people of other forms of religious and secular faith also became 'owners'. It was no longer necessary – or perhaps even desirable – to claim that the welfare state, the national health service or health care ethics were dependent upon Christian precepts. Instead, they are all projects that owed much to the intervention of Christians in the first place, but which now are *sui generis*.

A good illustration of these alternative understandings of secularisation is the different ways that Christian ethicists have reacted to Tom Beauchamp and James Childress' influential *Principles of Biomedical Ethics*.[4] Many Christian ethicists today are critical of the approach championed by Beauchamp and Childress – arguing that it marginalises Christian belief, privileges secular moral reasoning, and offers four arbitrary 'principles' for health care ethics (autonomy, justice, non-maleficence and beneficence) with inadequate meta-ethical justification. For them this is a clear example of secularisation in the first sense. Despite the fact that Childress still sees himself as a

---

[4] Tom L. Beauchamp and James F. Childress, *Principles of Biomedical Ethics* (Oxford and New York: Oxford University Press, 4th edn, 1994; it is this edition that will be used here).

Christian ethicist, they argue that he makes little attempt in his joint textbook with the secular philosopher Beauchamp to articulate (let alone defend) a distinctively Christian perspective. Instead he has in effect capitulated to the secularist.

In contrast, other Christian ethicists argue that this misunderstands the Beauchamp and Childress approach and unnecessarily polarises secular and religious ethicists concerned with issues in health care. Adopting the second understanding of secularisation, they applaud this attempt to find a basis for health care ethics that secular and religious people alike can use within a pluralistic society. They believe that it would be counterproductive to argue for an explicitly Christian version of health care ethics within such a society. Instead, a combination of Childress' implicit Christian perspective and Beauchamp's principled utilitarianism allows health care ethics to be genuinely inclusive and to mould the moral perceptions of health care workers and patients regardless of creed.

This brief account of health care ethics misses an obvious piece of evidence, namely that, despite the apparent triumph of secular philosophers and academic lawyers, theologians are still regularly included in the membership of national ethics committees concerned with science and medicine both in Britain and in the United States. Sometimes they are given the broader title of 'religious ethicist' but at other times the term 'theologian' is still used and (in Britain at least) it is in some instances a bishop who is included on such committees. At present, at least, there even seems to be some pressure on national ethics committees to be inclusive in this way.

Again, those holding these variant understandings of secularisation are likely to interpret this evidence quite differently. Holders of the first approach may well see this as an attempt by secular bodies to appear to be inclusive but without their making any serious concessions to the religiously committed. As long as it is just one religious ethicist who is included on a particular committee (as is usually the case), then there is little prospect that she/he will much affect the predominant secular discourse. More than that, there may be an implicit bargain that the religious ethicist adopts the secular discourse herself, or, if she does not, that she uses religious language simply to identify the idiosyncratic beliefs of variant religious minorities – in effect a sociological rather than theological use of distinctively religious language. Ironically, it may be sensitivity as much towards the beliefs of Jehovah's Witnesses as towards those of mainstream practising Jews, Christians or Muslims that such a religious ethicist is expected to represent as a member of such a committee.

Holders of the second approach to secularisation may well view this evidence differently. For them it perhaps represents a significant retreat from an ideologically secular understanding of health care ethics. Two rather different interpretations of 'secular' are present here. On one, health care ethics needs to be secular in order to be inclusive within a pluralist society, but, on the other, health care ethics becomes secular in order to eliminate specifically religious interpretations. The former includes both religion and non-religion, whereas the latter excludes religion. It is, of course, the former that is likely to appeal to followers of the second approach to secularisation. So, for them, the presence of a religious ethicist on a national ethics committee can be welcomed as a genuine attempt to be inclusive. This is not simply a sop to religious minorities but a recognition that a pluralistic society includes both those who are religious and those who are not.

Chapter 1 will argue that critical insights from Alasdair MacIntyre, Charles Taylor and John Hare can take this second approach considerably further. All three of these moral philosophers might argue that a pluralistic society should recognise that, not only do religious minorities need to be respected if such a society is to be genuinely inclusive, but that a number of crucial, but supposedly secular, moral notions in health care ethics have religious roots and may even make full sense only when these roots are explicitly acknowledged. Chapter 1 will explore this possibility under the broad heading of 'Moral gaps in secular health care ethics', first by examining some of the philosophical weaknesses of secular health care ethics and then by identifying some of the moral gaps that theologians might be encouraged to address.

MacIntyre, in particular, argues forcefully that there is an evident gap between his philosophical claims about virtue within communities and his sociological scepticism about actual communities within the modern world. He maintains that, if modernity is premised upon individual rationality, it founders upon incommensurable moral conflicts (the very conflicts that moral philosophy was supposed to resolve). A more post-modern vision is premised instead upon local communities shaping virtuous people, but it founders upon the seeming impossibility of achieving general assent today for returning to pre-modern communities. Moral fragmentation seems – so it appears in MacIntyre – to be inevitable.

The Beauchamp and Childress approach to health care ethics attempts to stave off this fragmentation by offering principles that can be justified by people holding quite different meta-ethical positions. In later editions of *Principles of Biomedical Ethics* the authors have also attempted to show that their approach is compatible with the increasingly influential virtue ethics approach to health care ethics. At best this seems to be a truce. As long as these principles can be upheld by different groups in medicine, albeit for very different reasons and, in addition, buffered by lawmakers, then they can be used to foster ethical discussion. Yet they remain vulnerable. And Taylor, despite being more committed to personal autonomy in ethics than MacIntyre, nevertheless believes that we are now in an age in which publicly accessible 'cosmic order of meanings' is an impossibility. All that we can rely upon today is 'personal resonance' – and that of course will vary from person to person.

John Hare identifies a third moral gap in secular ethics. Using Kantian arguments, he maintains that there is a gap between moral demands and a human propensity to selfishness. He argues that Kant himself was aware of this gap. The latter's categorical imperative made high moral demands. Yet his implicit Lutheranism also made him aware of humanity's tendency towards selfishness ... a selfishness that militated against the (unaided) human capacity to meet the demands of the categorical imperative.

Chapter 2 will explore how theologians have sought to make a distinctive contribution to health care ethics in the public forum, before addressing these three moral gaps: the gap between theoretical and actual moral communities; the gap between personal resonance and a shared understanding of cosmic order, and the gap between moral demands and human propensity to selfishness. Chapter 2 will identify a tension in public theology today between theological purists and theological realists and will then illustrate this tension within a specific area in health care ethics related to genetic science. A number of scientists would maintain emphatically that theology has nothing whatsoever to contribute in such an area. Even some religious scientists may be sceptical about any public role for theology on genetic issues. They may also be dismayed by what they regard as naïve theological utterances on specific scientific issues, especially on issues such as the genetic modification of food. In contrast, there is a growing theological literature which claims that a godless society is moving ever in a more destructive and irreligious direction, relegating (genetic) powers to itself that properly belong only to God.

It will be argued that there seems to be an increasing tension between those theologians who make sharply particularist claims (theological purists) and those who see only relative differences between Christian and secular thought (theological realists). The tension was apparent in the earliest phase of health care ethics – especially between pioneers such as Joseph Fletcher and Paul Ramsey in the United States[5] – but has become more pronounced today. Christian ethicists such as James Childress and Alastair Campbell contrast sharply with others such as Stanley Hauerwas and Gilbert Meilaender. Tristram Englehardt's, sometimes iconoclastic, work has been particularly important in exposing the issues involved in the tension. This chapter will take two books published in 1999 to illustrate it further, Michael Banner's *Christian Ethics and Contemporary Moral Problems* and Audrey R. Chapman's *Unprecedented Choices: Religious Ethics at the Frontiers of Genetic Science*. Since both Banner and Chapman are themselves involved as theologians on public bodies concerned with genetics and health care ethics, their work is directly relevant to this question about public theology. In theory, at least, they represent opposite positions on public theology, with Banner an enthusiastic Barthian, particularist and theological purist, and Chapman as more consensual, sympathetic to process theology and a theological realist. In practice, it will be seen that their differences are not so clear-cut. Both Chapman and Banner hold that Christian ethics has a distinctive critical function addressing moral gaps within the public forum. Whether this takes the form of questioning the sufficiency of autonomy as a moral principle or of pointing towards justice and concern

---

[5] See G. R. Dunstan's review of *On Moral Medicine* in *Journal of Medical Ethics*, 26:2 (2000), p. 77.

for the vulnerable (Chapman), or whether it entails reminding a pluralist society of the theological roots of many assumed values (Banner), there does seem to be a critical public role for the theologian.

This chapter will finally argue that public theology in health care ethics has a threefold critical role – criticising, deepening and widening the ethical debate in society at large. The deepening and widening aspects depend upon theistic and Christological assumptions, offering a vision for those who will hear of how things could be if all shared these assumptions and were committed to a Christian *eschaton*. Where this position differs from both Chapman and Banner is in expecting that the second and third functions can play a role in the direct work of public bodies concerned with ethics. It will be argued that the latter should remain sensitive to the beliefs of those who are religious within society at large, but that it is inappropriate in a pluralist context for them to adopt explicit theological beliefs themselves. Indeed, public bodies are likely to regard such explicit adoption not just as inappropriate but, given their fear of religious wars (strongly reinforced by September 11), as dangerously partisan. In addition, it is when public theologians imagine that, by virtue of being theologians, they have some special capacity for moral discernment on complex issues in bioscience that they can be most misleading. On this understanding, theologians do still need their secular colleagues: conversely, these colleagues may sometimes underestimate the motivation, commitment and depth which religious belonging and beliefs (or the heritage deriving from them) can still give people when making difficult ethical choices.

This dual perspective suggests that a cautious approach should be taken before claiming that theologians alone can close the three moral gaps identified in chapter 1. Continuing the discussion started in *Churchgoing and Christian Ethics*, religious communities do provide evidence of relative distinctiveness in the values/virtues held and practised by their participants. They supply at least partial evidence for the sort of virtuous communities envisaged by MacIntyre, but there is still a gap between their heritage and its actual implementation. Again, there is some evidence that even secular health care ethics contains implicit virtues derived from Judaeo-Christian communities (and also present within Islam) which may serve to narrow the gap between personal resonance and a shared understanding of cosmic order. Finally, there may be implicit residues of grace and faith within secular health care ethics that can narrow the gap between moral demands and a human propensity to selfishness. The suggestion made at this point is that virtues deriving from the specifically Judaeo-Christian heritage of the West (and resonating, at times, with virtues from Eastern religious heritages)[6] may yet implicitly inform secular health care ethics.

Chapter 3 will examine these implicit virtues, looking in detail at the healing stories in the Synoptic Gospels. It will be argued that, in the context of modern health care ethics, the 'miraculous' features of these stories (discussed in detail by Hugh Melinsky, from a tradition of theological realism, and by Colin Brown, from a more purist theological perspective) are less relevant than the virtues that shape them. It will also be argued that it would be anachronistic to jump from practices in these stories to modern medical practice. Following John Howard Kee and Gerd Theissen, this chapter will argue that the Synoptic healing stories should be understood in a first-century context before they are applied carefully to the twenty-first century. And, following John Pilch's biblical research using insights from medical anthropology, it will be argued that these stories have more to do with 'healing' than with 'cure' in the modern sense. A method will then be devised, derived from qualitative research in the social sciences, for identifying the most common virtues shaping the Synoptic healing stories.

Four virtues will be seen to be most distinctive. Compassion is the first of these, not because it is more frequent than the others but because it often comes at the beginning of a story. Occasionally the healing stories directly recount that Jesus was moved by compassion before healing someone. More often it is those to be healed or their friends/relatives who ask Jesus to show mercy or compassion. Sometimes the latter beg Jesus to respond. Compassion is also an important element within parables such as the merciful servant, the

---

[6] Although this book is a study in Christian ethics, I am certainly sympathetic to this wider religious resonance and will attempt to identify it *en passant*. But I must confess that I am a complete amateur in this area.

good Samaritan and the prodigal son, and is given by Mark as the initiating point for the feeding of both the four and the five thousand.

Care is a second distinctive virtue. This takes several forms. The most common of these forms is personal touching. An important part of many healing stories is Jesus touching the one to be healed, including touching those already identified in the story as 'unclean'. Many commentators identify this as ritual, even magical, action. However, from a perspective of healing, it may be viewed in more personal terms as the healer reaching out to care for the one who is to be healed but who has already been rejected by others as unclean. Another common form that care takes in the healing stories is anger. Sometimes Jesus appears to be angry at the illness or disability itself, sometimes Jesus 'sternly' warns those who have been healed not to tell others, but more often Jesus' anger is directed at religious author-ities who place their principles (especially about keeping the Sabbath) before helping the one who could be healed. Care in this double sense – Jesus caring through personal contact with the vulner-able and unclean and Jesus passionately caring that they should be healed – is a strong feature of these stories.

Faith is a third distinctive virtue. Jesus often notes the faith of those to be healed or of their friends/relatives, and, conversely, can do little to help when there is an absence of faith. A recurrent conclusion he draws is that 'your faith has made you well'. On two occasions – the centurion's servant and Canaanite woman – he particularly commends the faith of those who are not Jewish.

Reticence is a fourth virtue shaping the healing stories. A frequent end to healing stories in Mark, but also in places in Matthew (see especially Matt. 8 and 9) and Luke, is a command (in one place 'repeatedly') to the person healed to tell no one. Not surprisingly this feature has puzzled many biblical commentators. Even though Wrede's notion of the so-called messianic secret is now largely dis-counted, its shadow still remains in many commentaries. Viewed from a perspective of healing it may appear rather differently. There are frequent mentions in the Synoptic stories of the amazement of the crowds at the healings and alongside some of these are other indica-tions that Jesus was anxious to withdraw from the crowds. Viewed as miraculous 'signs' – an occasional observation in the Synoptic Gospels but far more explicit in the Fourth Gospel – Jesus' healings could appear simply to be a dramatic demonstration of who he really was. Yet viewed as the healer reaching out to the ill and disabled with compassion, care and faith, a command to reticence is perhaps less surprising. It is the one concerned to demonstrate miraculous signs who needs crowds, not the one who is most concerned to heal the vulnerable. There may also be another reason for reticence in the healing stories, namely the related virtue of humility. There are direct and indirect references in a number of the healing stories to 'power' and 'authority', set in a wider framework of teaching about the Kingdom of God. The healer who is conscious that it is finally God's power/rule that is at work in healing has good cause to feel personally humble.

Finally it will be seen in this chapter that, set in a wider context of religious ethics, all four of these virtues – compassion, care, faith and restraint – could be claimed by Judaism, Christianity and Islam alike. These virtues characterise Jesus as a Jew. According to Kee and Theissen, it is only their setting in a wider apocalyptic context within the Synoptic Gospels that differentiates them from contemporary Judaism. Again, although healing is not such a strong feature of the Qu'ran, these four virtues are very characteristic of the Qu'ran's sense of how good Muslims should behave: almost every *sura* begins with 'In the name of God, the Merciful, Compassionate'; followers of Jesus are specifically commended for their 'kindness' and compassion; care for the poor and vulnerable, especially through charitable giving, is a clear requirement for Muslims; faith is evident throughout the Qu'ran; and humility is required of those who remember that it is God who created them.

The next four chapters will seek to identify the relevance of each of these four virtues in turn for health care ethics today. They will argue that they are particularly relevant to the three moral gaps noted in chapter 1.

Chapter 4 will examine the role of compassion in health care ethics today. It will offer a two-fold critique, arguing that secular health care ethics has paid insufficient attention to compassion and that Christians have too often failed to put compassion before principled scruples.

The central problem in secular versions of health care ethics identified here is that, all too frequently, they overlook the starting point of good medical practice. For example, by launching straight into a discussion of the relative balance of the four principles (autonomy, justice, non-maleficence and beneficence), they forget to articulate the sense of compassion (understood as a response to the vulnerable and a determination to help them) that often motivates health care workers to act in the first place. Without compassion health care ethics can all too easily become cold and arid – 'clinical' in the pejorative sense.

The problem identified here with Christian versions of health care ethics is that too often they focus so solidly upon 'status of life' issues and then fail to show the sort of compassion exemplified by Jesus in the Synoptic Gospels. In particular, there is a recurring pattern in the Synoptics of Jesus allowing compassion to trump strongly held and principled scruples (such as not coming into physical contact with those who are impure or refraining from healing on the Sabbath).

A 'status of life' issue – namely whether or not it is right to withdraw nutrition and hydration from those totally lacking any cortical function – will be taken to illustrate how compassion can function with health care ethics. However, this will be deliberately balanced in later chapters by illustrations taken from issues more concerned with social justice in health care ethics. Within this particular chapter it will also lead to an exploration of the way the concept of 'covenant' – following Joseph Allen and William F. May – has generated important insights within this and other areas of health care ethics. This explicitly theological concept is premised upon God's faithfulness and loving-kindness to us and our consequent covenant to each other and to the rest of creation. However, it will finally be argued that within the public forum of a Western, pluralistic society the notion of 'compassion', properly understood, can perform a very similar but more inclusive role to that of covenant.

Chapter 5 will focus upon care within health care ethics today. The term 'care' is already widely used in secular medical contexts, for example in the term health care itself, in community care and care assistants. In the Synoptic healing stories Jesus both cared through personal and compassionate contact with the vulnerable and 'unclean' and passionately cared that they should be healed. This chapter will argue that an exploration of these stories, together with the related Lucan parables of the good or compassionate Samaritan and the prodigal son, reveals a critical tension on occasions between 'compassion' and 'care'. Compassion needs the structures of care to be effective and care needs compassion to direct it aright. But their aims are not always identical. Compassion for vulnerable individuals can sometimes be at odds with structures of care designed to bring lasting political or social change. This tension is already present in the Synoptic stories and parables and has important implications for health care ethics today.

Care, properly understood, also highlights the gap between moral demands and human propensity to selfishness. It is not always in the immediate interests of individuals to care for others or for the environment around them. And in an increasingly pluralistic society – that is a society in which there is a gap between personal resonance and a shared understanding of cosmic order – it is often difficult to reach agreement about what wider care entails.

Responses to those living with the growing pandemic of HIV/AIDS will be used to illustrate the various dimensions of the personal, compassionate and passionate Synoptic vision of care. After an initial phase of denial and denouncement, Christian responses to those living with HIV/AIDS have slowly become more compassionate and caring. There are strong parallels here with the Synoptic Jesus' response to those living with leprosy. However, HIV/AIDS today can sometimes involve a sharp dichotomy between a proper concern for the individuals living with the virus and public health attempts to limit, or even halt, its spread. The Christian ethicist David Hollenbach's analysis of the creative tension between individualistic notions of tolerance, on the one hand, and the common good, on the other, will be used to understand care in the global context of HIV/AIDS better.

Chapter 6 will explore the role of faith in health care ethics today. Faith or trust is important at a number of different levels. In the Synoptic healing stories 'faith' is already quite varied: sometimes it refers to the faith of the person to be healed; sometimes it is the faith of the relatives or friends; sometimes it appears to be faith in Jesus as healer; sometimes it seems to be faith in God; sometimes faith appears to be belief; sometimes it seems rather to be trust; sometimes it is the faith of fellow Jews; sometimes that of Gentiles. It is also varied in health care ethics today. The recent powerful Reith and

Gifford Lectures of Onora O'Neill will be examined carefully to show that some level of 'trust' between patients and medical professionals is vital. Yet, so O'Neill argues, despite huge advances in modern medicine and a careful audit culture designed to enhance trust, public suspicion rather than trust is now all too apparent. This chapter will also examine the claims of the secular sociologist Paul Halmos, a generation earlier, that 'faith' is essential to the work of health care professionals themselves.

Particularly important in this chapter is the growing empirical evidence that there is a connection between religious belonging and health. This suggests that religious belonging is a significant (but often ignored) independent variable in promoting physical and psychological health. The recent work of Harold Koenig and Byron Johnson has examined this empirical evidence in enormous detail. There is still much debate about the causal factors involved here and sometimes bold claims have been made that are problematic at both a methodological and theological level. However, this chapter will argue that motivation and critical depth are crucial. People with a strong religious involvement are more likely than others to have a sense of purpose in life and to be altruistic (as shown earlier in *Churchgoing and Christian Ethics*). In turn, such motivation may have important implications for physical and psychological health. While healing is obviously possible without such faith being made explicit, elements of it are likely to be implicit within many healing contexts. It is also at this level that the moral gap between the demand of moral duty and human propensity to selfishness can be narrowed. For the medical professional, especially when grounded in a worshipping community, faith in this third sense offers a powerful source of motivation to act selflessly. For the patient such a community can also narrow the gap between personal resonance and a shared understanding of cosmic order.

Chapter 7 will explore the role of reticence or humility within health care ethics today. It will be argued that medical professionals can claim too much and patients can demand too much. Both are damaging to health care and distort health care ethics. The careful account of different virtues provided by Jean Porter will be examined to see how humility relates to compassionate care and faith – a balance concerned with the interrelation of other-regarding and self-regarding virtues. Both sort of virtues, she argues, are essential to a full account of ethics. In the context of exaggerated claims about the role of genetic science in modern medicine, it will be maintained that humility (alongside compassionate care and faith) is extremely important.

Perhaps the most intractable area of health care ethics is that of rationing or prioritising. Finding an ethical way of allocating scarce medical resources – given modern advances in medical science and an apparently limitless patient demand – has proved extremely difficult. The, finally inconclusive, work of John Butler in this area will be explored in some detail. This leads to the suggestion that humility – in the sense of medical professionals not claiming too much and patients not demanding too much – may have a more important role than Butler suggests if the difficult ethical issues involved in health care rationing are at least to be reduced. Humility may also have an important relationship to the faith of medical professionals and/or patients. This chapter will then examine critically the more ambitious theological claims made in Tristram Engelhardt and Mark Cherry's collection *Allocating Scarce Medical Resources: Roman Catholic Perspectives.*

In conclusion, this book will argue that, properly understood, the four distinctively religious virtues of compassion, care, faith and humility complement rather than conflict with the four bioethics principles of autonomy, justice, non-maleficence and beneficence. It is right that compassion should impel medical professionals to care for those in need and that, in turn, care should involve both caring about and caring for those who become patients. A proper understanding of the relationship between medical professionals and their patients also requires them to pay attention to non-maleficence, beneficence and the autonomy of these patients – and, in turn, for patients also to respect their autonomy. Faith is involved in some sense in the healing relationship between both parties and, for some, also between them and God. Justice is also an essential consideration in the broader context of health in society at large. And finally humility should restrain both medical professionals from making exaggerated claims and patients from making selfish demands.

CHAPTER I

Moral gaps in secular health care ethics

Within the secular post-Enlightenment tradition following Kant moral agency was characteristically perceived as being independent of religion and based instead upon autonomous rationality alone. Thus, the individual makes moral choices and decisions based solely upon rational criteria that are available to all competent, rational agents (whether they are themselves privately religious, as Kant was, or not). Alasdair MacIntyre's seminal *After Virtue* challenged this understanding of moral agency. At a negative level, he argued that moral philosophy – the discipline concerned with autonomous, rational criteria in moral thinking – has been unable to deliver indisputable rational criteria or universally agreed moral decisions. Incommensurable differences remain on key moral issues such as abortion or justice both within the general public and (especially and most significantly) among experts in moral philosophy. At a positive level, he argued that virtues moulded by moral and often religious communities are essential to an adequate understanding of moral agency. Charles Taylor's *Sources of the Self* also challenged a purely secular understanding of moral agency. Although more committed than MacIntyre to a notion of autonomy within moral agency, he nevertheless argued that moral reasoning cannot be properly under-stood without acknowledging the long history of moral concepts within specific and typically religious communities.

MORAL GAP ONE

A central part of MacIntyre's critique of moral philosophy is that it makes claims for secular reasoning that it is unable to deliver. Thus in the name of the Enlightenment the discipline has tended to claim that it alone, unlike theological ethics, can resolve moral dilemmas in the public realm. Moral reasoning without any divine revelation can be a universal means of reaching moral conclusions. Whereas theology divides people, moral philosophy can unite them: through the Enlightenment understanding of morality we have been delivered from the bitter religious warfare that characterised Europe during the sixteenth and seventeenth centuries. Decision-making based upon moral philosophy offers the prospect of agreement across cultural and ideological divisions.

After Virtue subjects such claims to a detailed critique. There is, so the book argues, a clear gap between such claims and their attainment. Within moral philosophy there are very evident and unresolved differences between, for example, deontologists and utilitarians. These differences become apparent as soon as recent debates are examined about issues such as the rightness of abortion or the nature of justice in society. MacIntyre argues that these are not differences that are yet to be resolved but that are capable eventually of resolution when moral philosophy is used properly. Rather he maintains that they are actually differences that are incommensurable in terms of post-Enlightenment moral philosophy.

So the differences between pro-life and pro-choice factions in the abortion debate are not, so MacIntyre argues, resolvable in terms of post-Enlightenment moral philosophy. All too often contesting rights of the fetus, on the one hand, or of the woman, on the other, are simply asserted by the different factions without any prospect of rational resolution between them. Even elegant attempts to resolve this contestation – notably that of Ronald Dworkin[1] – have so far failed to convince either faction. Of course particular power groups within society can ensure that, in the absence of intellectual agreement, one of these factions prevails. In reality this has now happened in much secular health care ethics within the West in favour of the pro-choice faction. So, although there is still a widespread belief that it is right to have a conscience clause allowing health care professionals opposed to abortion not to take a direct part in providing abortions, the same professionals are nevertheless still obliged to refer

---

[1] Ronald Dworkin, *Life's Dominion: an Argument about Abortion and Euthanasia* (London: Harper Collins, 1993).

women requesting an abortion to other professionals who are not opposed. At best this is a conscience clause allowing professionals to opt out of direct action on abortion but not to opt out of abortion provision altogether (akin, perhaps, to ambulance service on the front line in the First World War for exemplary pacifists rather than incarceration for thoroughgoing pacifists).

Again, both MacIntyre and Taylor argue that a central weakness of much recent moral philosophy is 'atomised individualism'. It is all too often assumed that moral conclusions are typically reached by individuals through a series of logical steps without reference to others or to tradition until they make a moral decision. The focus here is upon the self as a self-contained island and upon moral decisions reached by an internalised process of logical deduction, as if individuals were not actually part of wider communities embedded in history and tradition. Taylor's *Sources of the Self* seeks to show at length that this is a very impoverished understanding of the moral self. Yet, ironically, it is still an understanding that is implicit within much discussion of autonomy and decision-making in health care ethics.[2]

In contrast to 'atomised individualism' MacIntyre returns to the moral tradition of virtue ethics and points to the role of moral communities in shaping virtuous individuals. Within this tradition individuals are trained in virtues within local communities so that, when faced with ethical dilemmas, they do not approach them *de novo* as isolated individuals but as members of communities and as heirs to long-standing sources of moral wisdom. Such individuals depend less upon secular rationality than upon deeply ingrained virtuous habits to resolve moral dilemmas. On this understanding of health care ethics – an understanding which is beginning to receive more serious discussion – the primary task of the discipline is to identify virtues which should guide and shape health care professionals and patients alike.

Herein lies a central problem. MacIntyre himself is highly sceptical about whether Western society is again capable of having a unified moral vision. Having deconstructed the universal claims of moral

[2] See Gordon M. Stirrat and Robin Gill, 'Autonomy in Medical Ethics after O'Neill', *Journal of Medical Ethics*, 31:2 (2005), pp. 127–30.

philosophy, he sees only fragmented and changing moral communities in the Western world. He points to the need for a new moral community, but offers little hope that it is actually still possible for any moral community to gain widespread acceptance. At most, presumably, a series of fragmented communities can bring their virtues to modern medicine, but without any expectation that everyone can accept them.

MacIntyre's sharp scepticism may in the end be his most enduring legacy. Principally there is his scepticism about the ability of atomistic, liberal individualism, or of purely secular rationalism, to resolve moral issues adequately. This scepticism has taken several forms. Sometimes it is philosophical, with MacIntyre noting the inability of rival groups of deontologists and utilitarians to agree among or between themselves, despite their separate claims to be able to resolve moral issues on universal rational grounds. Sometimes it is sociological, with him calling attention to the levels of moral disagreement apparent in pluralistic modern societies and a consequent inability to agree upon common virtues. Sometimes it is historical, with him contending that the historical embeddedness of moral ideas is frequently ignored and misunderstood in modern society – most people are no longer aware of the origins of their own ideas.

Naturally, since the original publication of *After Virtue* in 1981, MacIntyre has faced many critics. One of the most seminal collections of his critics was published in 1994 with the inevitable title *After MacIntyre*.[3] Some of the authors in this collection seek to defend post-Enlightenment liberalism and utilitarianism against MacIntyre's intellectual onslaught. Others correct his Aristotelianism and increasing Thomism. And others again simply seek to clarify his arguments. At the end of the collection MacIntyre responds.

The group that receives the sharpest criticism from MacIntyre consists understandably of those still writing within the parameters of the 'Enlightenment project'. Robert Wokler believes that MacIntyre's paradigm is too univocal and exaggerated: it is highly selective and lacks sufficient historical nuance. For Wokler the 'Enlightenment

---

[3] John Horton and Susan Mendus (eds.), *After MacIntyre: Critical Perspectives on the Work of Alasdair MacIntyre* (Oxford and Notre Dame, IN: Polity Press and University of Notre Dame Press, 1994).

project' at the heart of MacIntyre's recent writings is 'profoundly
misleading'.[4] At the end of his essay he even teases MacIntyre with
the suggestion that on the latter's precepts the eighteenth-century
electors were right to deny David Hume the Edinburgh Chair of
Moral Philosophy. Paul Kelly similarly subjects MacIntyre's dis-
missal of utilitarianism to a spirited critique and Philip Pettit,
Stephen Mulhall and Andrew Mason variously offer critical examinations of aspects of his critique of liberalism. In response MacIntyre
argues that post-Enlightenment liberalism, when viewed in all its
complexity, faces very serious problems of incommensurability:

> Liberalism . . . as a form of social life, is partly constituted by its continuing
> internal debates between rival incommensurable points of view. In this it
> resembles many other social and cultural traditions. Each one of those
> points of view has itself been elaborated within a tradition of enquiry
> constituted by agreements upon shared standards. So that characteristically,
> at least up to a certain point, within each tradition there has been by its own
> standards progress in problem-solving, while in the conflicts between tradi-
> tions there has been no rational progress at all. Incommensurability has
> precluded it.[5]

In his contribution to *After MacIntyre*, Charles Taylor adopts a
characteristically both/and approach: both agreeing with MacIntyre's
Aristotelian emphasis upon virtues within historic communities and
valuing the post-Enlightenment stress upon individual autonomy:

> MacIntyre . . . tends to take modern society at the face value of its own
> dominant theories, as heading for runaway atomism and break-up. He
> speaks at times of a society organized around 'emotivist' understandings
> of ethics. I, on the other hand, frankly lean in the other direction. I think
> that we are far more 'Aristotelian' than we allow, that hence our practice is
> in some significant way less based on pure disengaged freedom and atom-
> ism than we realize.[6]

MacIntyre bluntly dismisses this approach as incoherent and
remains unconvinced that it is possible to combine these two

---

[4] Robert Wokler, 'Projecting the Enlightenment', in Horton and Mendus, *After MacIntyre*,
   p. 111.
[5] Alasdair MacIntyre, 'A Partial Response to my Critics', in Horton and Mendus, *After
   MacIntyre*, p. 292.
[6] Charles Taylor, 'Justice after Virtue', in Horton and Mendus, *After MacIntyre*, p. 22.

philosophical traditions. He is, though, more sympathetic towards his explicitly Thomist critics, such as John Haldane and Janet Coleman. His own preference is for Aristotle, since he focuses upon 'the apprenticeship to any tradition-constituted practice and the boundaries across traditions', whereas his Thomist critics are more concerned with 'the nature of rational justification and of that attainment of truth which constitutes the telos of rational enquiry'.[7] In effect, he maintains, these are different spheres rather than incompatible approaches. Of course he did not have the space in this response to argue his position more fully. However I am not aware that he has yet argued it adequately elsewhere, demonstrating just how he meshes his own position of moral practice, moulded and sustained in historically changing communities, with his increasing sympathy towards Thomism.

David Fergusson expresses similar doubts. In his contribution to *New Studies in Christian Ethics*, Fergusson spends much longer than myself on MacIntyre, reviewing in the process a much wider range of his recent writings. Fergusson argues positively that 'MacIntyre's work is of major significance in reintroducing the discourse of the Christian faith to moral philosophy at the highest level.'[8] Nevertheless, he still sees 'theological deficiencies' even in his most recent work. For example, Fergusson cites MacIntyre's remarks about grace being able to correct faulty moral reasoning and concludes:

The Christian ethos of the moral life is not adequately captured in such remarks. The way in which moral activity within the Christian life is determined by a range of conceptions including the divine command, obedience, grace, justification, the body of Christ, sanctification, and response to God's action *extra nos* seem somehow to be missing. These shape not only the moral perception of the Christian, but also the moral seriousness, commitment, and motivation which characterise a life of faith.[9]

But this is a point for another context. What is interesting here is MacIntyre's negative thesis, his radical scepticism … namely, that

---

[7] Alasdair MacIntyre, 'A Partial Response to my Critics', in Horton and Mendus, *After MacIntyre*, p. 300.

[8] David Fergusson, *Community, Liberalism and Christian Ethics* (Cambridge: Cambridge University Press, 1998), p. 137.

[9] Fergusson, *Community*, p. 136.

he identifies a crucial moral gap in secular moral philosophy arising from what he sees as the issue of incommensurability within late-modern, secular society. Expressed differently, it is the gap between theoretical and actual moral communities.

MORAL GAP TWO

Charles Taylor's influential *Sources of the Self* identifies a second major moral gap. He believes that we are now in an age in which publicly accessible 'cosmic order of meanings' is an impossibility.[10] All that we can rely upon today is 'personal resonance' – and that of course will vary from person to person. He likens us to a crew of car mechanics in a pit-stop, each with four thumbs and with only a very hazy grasp of the wiring used in modern racing cars. We have become thoroughly confused today about the sources of the self that constitute modern notions of identity. Taylor traces, for example, the way that naturalism and utilitarianism have contributed to this confusion, creating for many a severe tension:

> what remains is an extremely important fact about modern moral consciousness: a tension between the affirmation of ordinary life, to which we moderns are strongly drawn, and some of our most important moral distinctions. Indeed, it is too simple to speak of a tension. We are in conflict, even confusion, about what it means to affirm ordinary life. What for some is the highest affirmation is for others blanket denial. Think of the utilitarian attack on orthodox Christianity; then of Dostoyevsky's attack on utilitarian utopian engineering. For those who are not firmly aligned on one side or the other of an ideological battle, this is the source of a deep uncertainty. We are as ambivalent about heroism as we are about the value of the workaday goals that it sacrifices. We struggle to hold onto a vision of the incomparably higher, while being true to the central modern insights about the values of ordinary life. We sympathize with both the hero and the anti-hero; and we dream of a world in which one could be in the same act both.[11]

One practical way of resolving this tension/confusion is to resort to mundane procedures in an attempt to counter this serious deficiency.

---

[10] Charles Taylor, *Sources of the Self: the Making of the Modern Identity* (Cambridge, MA: Harvard University Press, 1989), p. 512.

[11] Taylor, *Sources*, p. 24.

This is the approach deliberately adopted by Tom Beauchamp and James Childress in their highly influential *Principles of Biomedical Ethics.*[12] They identify their approach as 'practical ethics':

The term *practical* refers to the use of ethical theory and methods of analysis to examine moral problems, practices, and policies in several areas, including the professions and public policy. Often no straightforward movement from theory or principles to particular judgments is possible in these contexts, although general reasons, principles, or even ideals can play some role in evaluating conduct and establishing policies. Theory and principles are typically invoked only to help develop action-guides, which are also further shaped by paradigm cases of appropriate behavior, empirical data, and the like, together with reflection on how to put these influential sources into the most coherent whole.[13]

Although they come from very different intellectual and spiritual traditions – Beauchamp from a secular utilitarian tradition and Childress from a Quaker tradition – they do have a shared concern to develop 'general moral action-guides for use in the biomedical fields', based upon a tension between the four principles of autonomy, non-maleficence, beneficence and justice. The latter offers, so they argue, a rational basis for discussing health care ethics in a pluralistic society. Indeed, their approach has successfully allowed secular and religious ethicists to contribute on an equal footing in health care ethics without being paralysed by their meta-ethical differences.[14] Although it does not explicitly adopt the Beauchamp and Childress approach, the British Medical Association's authoritative *Medical Ethics Today*[15] is in reality based upon a very similar 'practical ethics' approach. In the context of the public forum of a Western, pluralistic society, it is difficult to see how the BMA could have adopted any other approach. As the doctors' trade union in Britain, the BMA does also need to represent adequately its own increasingly pluralistic and multi-cultural constituency.

[12] Tom L. Beauchamp and James F. Childress, *Principles of Biomedical Ethics* (Oxford and New York: Oxford University Press, 4th edn, 1994).
[13] Beauchamp and Childress, *Principles*, p. 4.
[14] See, for example, R. Gillon (ed.), *Principles of Health Care Ethics* (London: Wiley, 1985).
[15] British Medical Association Ethics Department, *Medical Ethics Today* (London: BMJ Books, 2004).

Nevertheless, such a 'practical ethics' approach does not actually resolve Charles Taylor's point that we no longer share a vision of 'cosmic order of meaning'. For example, within health care ethics, it is painfully obvious that in Western, pluralistic societies today we cannot even agree upon a notion of 'health': for some it is concerned narrowly with an absence of physical 'disease' (itself a term with cultural variants), whereas for others it is concerned with wider well-being (a term with meta-ethical variants) and for others still with physical, mental and spiritual health (now with metaphysical variants). And when notions of 'health' and 'disease' are used in such contentious areas as involuntary psychiatric treatment, public disagreement abounds. As William Fulford argues, in this area especially 'the very classification of diseases, and with it medical diagnosis, depends not just on the facts but on the construction that is placed on the facts'.[16] Or to apply it to the area of modern warfare, it is often extremely difficult if not impossible to get opposing factions to agree about how just-war theory actually applies to them. For example, one side may see a particular recourse to arms as being a legitimate struggle for liberation, whereas the opposing side may see it instead as an act of terrorism.

Another way to resolve the tension/confusion is again to resort simply to coercion. Taylor is well aware of this possibility and warns against it, using the distribution of goods as an illustration:

The members of our society would expect goods to be distributed according to desert, understood in terms of mutual indebtedness in the pursuit of the common good. Let us call this distribution MD. The Rawlsian would hold that to live up to the demands of our highest good we ought to adopt distribution TD. TD conflicts, let us say, with MD. What ought we to do? The generally accepted answer is that there is no problem. If we think that Rawls's notion of the good is right, then TD is right, and so MD must be wrong. But my point is that this does not follow. The fact that TD represents what we ought to live with to conform to the best in us does not show at all that MD also does not correspond to legitimate expectations, that A having risked or sacrificed so much for the common good does really deserve more, that there would be a real wrong (yes, an injustice) involved in

[16] K. W. M. Fulford, 'No More Medical Ethics', in K. W. M. Fulford, Grant R. Gillett and Janet Martin Soskice (eds.), *Medicine and Moral Reasoning* (Cambridge: Cambridge University Press, 1994), p. 194.

denying this to A against his will. Of course, in a society made up totally of convinced Rawlsians, A would happily forgo this entitlement; but if this is not our case, TD would have to be enforced against his will, in violation of his sense of right: and in this case, it would constitute an injustice. We have a dilemma on our hands.[17]

For Taylor the central dilemma for modernity is the moral gap between personal resonance and a shared understanding of cosmic order. Because we no longer have the latter (even secular forms of naturalism and utilitarianism have failed to become universally convincing), we find our conflicting senses of personal resonance deeply problematic.

We do, indeed, have a dilemma on our hands. At the beginning of his *The Foundations of Bioethics*, Tristram Engelhardt summarises this dilemma forcefully:

Rather than philosophy being able to fill the void left by the collapse of the hegemony of Christian thought in the West, philosophy has shown itself to be many competing philosophies and philosophical ethics. The attempt to sustain a secular equivalent of Western Christian monotheism through the disclosure of a unique moral and metaphysical account of reality has fragmented into a polytheism of perspectives with its chaos of moral diversity and its cacophony of numerous competing moral narratives. This circumstance as a sociological condition, reflecting our epistemological limitations, defines postmodernity. Secular rationality appears triumphant. But it has become many rationalities. It is not clear whether it can give moral or metaphysical orientation.[18]

MORAL GAP THREE

Within a detailed discussion of Kantian ethics in his significant, but less well-known, book *The Moral Gap: Kantian Ethics, Human Limits and God's Assistance*, John Hare suggests a third major moral gap. He argues that this is the gap that arises from Kant's high moral demand for individuals combined with his belief that everyone has a propensity not to follow this demand. Specifically, the high moral demand

---

[17] Charles Taylor, 'Justice after Virtue', in Horton and Mendus, *After MacIntyre*, pp. 39–40.
[18] H. Tristram Engelhardt Jr, *The Foundations of Bioethics* (New York: Oxford University Press, 2nd edn, 1996), p. 5.

that all people should always behave morally in ways that are universalisable is in clear tension with their propensity to selfishness. This selfishness may take several forms:

There are failures of self-deception. For example, I may magnify the intensity of my own preferences, so that they outweigh the preferences of others in the moral calculus; or I may cloak self-interest in the disguise of normative principles with the appearance of objectivity. There are failures of patience, where I am so convinced of the merit of my cause that I cannot even listen to the claims of another person. There are, above all, failures of impartiality, in which I do understand the preferences of another, and I do adopt them as hypothetical preferences of my own for the situation in which I would be that person, but I then refuse to give those hypothetical preferences equal weight with my preferences for the actual situation in which I occupy my actual role.[19]

For Kant, Hare argues, this gap was particularly acute precisely because he believed that 'ought' implies 'can': if it is not the case that people can live by the moral demand, then it cannot be the case that they ought to do so. Hare is unconvinced by secular strategies designed to reduce this moral gap. The first seeks to reduce the moral demand itself (perhaps moral demands need not be universalisable) and the second exaggerates our natural propensities (perhaps humans really are not selfish after all). Both of these strategies have also been used at times in health care ethics: if the moral demands in health care ethics are sufficiently low then we should be able to attain them, or if we can assume that all health care professionals and patients will act selflessly then we can keep the demands high.

Rejecting such strategies, Hare sets out to explore how Christian faith might be able to bridge this moral gap. He argues that academic philosophy has persistently underestimated Kant's Christianity:

His system does not work unless he is seen as genuinely trying to 'make room for faith'. Failure to see this has led to heroic measures, either excising portions of text as not properly 'critical', or attributing his views to a desire to appease the pious sentiments of his faithful manservant. What is true of Kant is also true of Descartes, Hobbes, Leibniz, and even Hume. We are given a reading of modern philosophy that leads from its birth in the new

---

[19] John Hare, *The Moral Gap* (Oxford: Clarendon Paperbacks, Oxford University Press, 1997), p. 25.

science of the sixteenth century to its maturation in the death of God and the death of metaphysics ... It is no doubt tempting, if you cannot take Christianity seriously yourself, to interpret your favourite philosophers as sharing this distaste; but it leads to a distortion of the texts.[20]

In contrast to such secular accounts of philosophy, Hare argues that a notion of God's assistance, or 'divine supplementation', was essential to Kant's dual way of resolving this third moral gap (i.e. between the moral demand on us and our natural capacity to live by it). The first way involved the belief that 'Heaven will find the means to make up our deficiency', whereas the second was as follows:

It is a person's faith that her future happiness does not require her to give up the attempt to lead a morally good life. This faith bridges the gap also, because it makes possible for her to combine her built-in desire for her own happiness with a commitment to morality. If she does have this second kind of moral faith, does she still need the first? She does, because morality requires its followers not only to pursue both duty and happiness, but to give duty priority over their other commitments. The first kind of moral faith allows her to believe that she can give morality this kind of priority, and that this revolution of the will has actually been accomplished in her.[21]

Hare is careful not to claim that Kant had a fully developed Christian theology of grace. He also distances himself from Stanley Hauerwas' typical position where Kant 'is lumped into "the Enlightenment" without remainder, and the Enlightenment is charged with casting off tradition and community and narrative and the virtues'.[22] Nonetheless, together with MacIntyre and Taylor, Hare is concerned to question the easy secular assumption that ethics in the public forum need pay no attention whatsoever to theology. Each of these three moral philosophers (despite their strongly held internal differences) is convinced that Western philosophy has serious moral gaps and ignores its Christian heritage at its peril.

RESPONSES

This growing conviction has been highly influential among Christian ethicists, suggesting a number of new assumptions. The first is that

[20] Hare, *Moral Gap*, pp. 2–3.   [21] Hare, *Moral Gap*, p. 69.   [22] Hare, *Moral Gap*, p. 35.

late modernity is characterised by global pluralism rather than by secularity. For John Milbank modern secularism is not a neutral platform for examining the world, but itself a form of ideology (Milbank even argues that it is a form of 'implicit' theology).[23] The second is that, within this global pluralism, differing and sometimes competing religious communities abide and continue to contribute to moral agency. And the third is that such religious communities properly understood – and despite their internal differences – do still have a significant role to play in the public forum even within secular democracies.

A good illustration of this is the extent to which religious ethicists and religious leaders both in the United States and in the United Kingdom, and more widely within Europe, have recently been involved in public discussions of the morality of military action following September 11 and the morality of novel scientific areas such as that of stem cell research. As noted in the Introduction, it is now a feature of many national committees established to consider such moral issues that they regularly include a religious ethicist, alongside secular philosophers and lawyers. Politicians within both the United States and the United Kingdom are very wary of basing public policy upon any specific religious teaching (even within the Republic of Ireland such an approach is no longer popular). Not the least of the fears is the risk of alienating other religious minorities within their respective countries. So there is little prospect that public theologians today will ever be able to have the sort of political influence once commanded by Reinhold Niebuhr. Nonetheless, there does seem to be a growing recognition today that religious groups may have a distinctive contribution to make to the well-being of society at large.

Lisa Cahill makes a further important point. Even if it is the case that national committees concerned with health care ethics once included more theologians than they typically do today, such committees are by no means the only available forum for public theology. She argues that John Evans[24] 'and other critics of the secularisation of

---

[23] John Milbank, *Theology and Social Theory* (Oxford: Blackwell, 1990).

[24] John H. Evans, *Play God? Human Genetic Engineering and the Rationalization of Public Bioethical Debate* (Chicago: Chicago University Press, 2002).

bioethics keep their gaze so firmly fixed on governmental bodies such as public commissions, regulatory agencies, and legislatures'[25] that they overlook other forms of religiously inspired local and global activism. Using insights from Michel Foucault's analysis of how modern 'discourse' about sex co-opts everyone discussing sex into the belief that their sexuality is under illegitimate constraints that must be thrown off, she argues:

One might conclude the same about the supposed 'marginalization' of theology in bioethics, taking note of the number of papers and articles that have dealt with the phenomenon in the past fifteen or more years. The parallel with Foucault's analysis of sexual 'repression' is especially striking, in light of the never-ending advocacy of many churches, religious groups, and theologians for 'pro-life' causes. The prevailing discourse has managed virtually to equate 'religious bioethics' with such advocacy, constructing it as a public danger, even while insisting on its marginality. An important corollary is that the 'official' discourse also establishes the bioethics issues that will be central to public policy ... the focal issue is undoubtedly the protection of autonomy by procedural guarantees of informed consent. Meanwhile, religion is framed as entirely preoccupied with 'status of life' issues.[26]

For Cahill this produces a thoroughly distorted public perception of religious activism. In particular, it overlooks extensive local and global religious activism concerned with issues of justice and social change in health care provision. She gives as examples the considerable work done by Christian ethicists on distributive justice in health care resource allocation[27] (chapter 7 will return to this issue) and the active involvement of church groups and other NGOs in pressurising major pharmaceutical companies to loosen their patents of anti-retroviral drugs for those living with HIV/AIDS in sub-Saharan Africa (chapter 5 will return to this). She believes that 'for theological bioethics to reassert and extend its authority in emerging global practices of research and health care distribution, especially

---

[25] Lisa Sowle Cahill, 'Bioethics, Theology, and Social Change', *Journal of Religious Ethics*, 31:3 (2003), p. 369.
[26] Cahill, 'Bioethics', pp. 370–1.
[27] For example, see H. Tristram Engelhardt Jr, and Mark J. Cherry (eds.), *Allocating Scarce Medical Resources: Roman Catholic Perspectives* (Washington, DC: Georgetown University Press, 2002).

genomics, it will be necessary to take the "preferential option for the poor" beyond rhetorical or abstract conflicts with countervailing social norms'.[28]

One recent, striking example of theologically inspired activism, focused upon public policy and with important implications for health care ethics, is the Family, Religion and Culture Project directed from Chicago University by Don Browning. Books published as a result of this project have attempted to give an overview of the social and theological debate about the family in modern America. At the heart of the Family, Religion and Culture Project is a conviction that the family should be defended robustly by Christians, despite the fact that in the name of the Bible it has often been distorted in the past. In the foundation book for the series, *From Culture Wars to Common Ground: Religion and the American Family Debate*,[29] the authors argue that the fundamental family issue of our time may be how to retain and honour the intact family without turning it into an object of idolatry and without retaining the inequalities of power, status and privilege ensconced in its earlier forms. Using extensive social statistics they argue that in America today one out of two marriages ends in divorce and almost one in three children is born outside marriage, with disastrous consequences for the health and welfare of these children. Yet the United States is still a country of relatively high religious attendance and over two-thirds of all marriages take place in churches and synagogues. Second and even third marriages regularly take place in Christian churches in the United States and increasingly within the United Kingdom as well. Those writing for the Project are well aware of these facts when they seek to defend what they term the 'intact' family – by which they mean families in which children are brought up by both of their biological parents. Not wishing in any way to discriminate against other families, they still believe that it is vital for religious communities to encourage intact families, if necessary with help from the law, if the health and welfare of children are properly to be protected. Thus, they articulate a position which in the

---

[28] Cahill, 'Bioethics', p. 391.
[29] Don Browning, Bonnie Miller-McLemore, Pamela Couture, Bernie Lyon and Robert Franklin, *From Culture Wars to Common Ground* (Louisville, KY: Westminster/John Knox, 1997).

next chapter I will identify as 'theological realism' (in contrast to those theological purists who do wish to discriminate against 'other families'). It is also a position that is considerably at odds with the prevailing secular consensus that tends to regard the intact family as just one (possibly anachronistic) option.

Another approach, which I set out at length in *Churchgoing and Christian Ethics*,[30] is based less upon a moral campaign than upon an attempt to assess in social scientific terms just how significant religious factors are in moral agency. Using extensive international data from social attitude questionnaires, I test whether claimed religious behaviour or belief has any relationship to more general moral attitudes or action. What emerges is that the religiously active are indeed distinctive in their attitudes and behaviour. Some of their attitudes do change over time, especially on issues such as sexuality, and there are obvious moral disagreements between different groups of churchgoers in a number of areas. Nonetheless, there are broad patterns of belief, teleology and altruism that distinguish those who are religiously active from those who are not. For example, Christian churchgoers have, in addition to their distinctive theistic and Christocentric beliefs, a strong sense of moral order and concern for other people. They are more likely than others to be involved in voluntary service and to see overseas charitable giving as important. They are more hesitant about euthanasia and capital punishment and more concerned about the family and civic order than other people. None of these differences is absolute. The values, virtues, moral attitudes and behaviour of churchgoers are shared by many other people as well. The distinctiveness of churchgoers is real but relative.

This evidence is consonant with Alasdair MacIntyre's *After Virtue*. There he recognises that, even in pluralistic American society, there are still religious communities – Catholic Irish, Orthodox Greeks and Orthodox Jews – which are relatively less fragmented. Yet, 'even however in such communities the need to enter into public debate enforces participation in the cultural *mélange* in the search for a common stock of concepts and norms which all may enjoy and to

---

[30] Robin Gill, *Churchgoing and Christian Ethics* (Cambridge: Cambridge University Press, 1999).

which all may appeal . . . in search of what, if my argument is correct, is a chimaera'. This produces a curious mixture of historically and culturally contingent communities misguidedly searching for moral consensus. MacIntyre argues that 'moral philosophies, however they may aspire to achieve more than this, always do articulate the morality of some particular social and cultural standpoint'. As a result, modern, pluralistic societies cannot hope to achieve moral consensus. Rather, 'it is in its historical encounter that any given point of view establishes or fails to establish its rational superiority relative to its particular rivals in some specific contexts'.[31] A pattern, then, is to be expected: moral agency within religious communities today may well be distinctive, but may still overlap at many points with that of 'secular' communities.

In *Churchgoing and Christian Ethics* I discuss whether a causal relationship can be established between churchgoing and the distinctive virtues that regular churchgoers hold to a greater degree than other people. The strongest evidence for such a relationship involves comparing the responses of two groups of non-churchgoers – the one originally brought up going to church almost every week and the other never going in childhood at all. This suggests that the effects of involuntary churchgoing as a child can still be traced in the relative strength of the Christian beliefs of adult non-churchgoers. Compared with non-churchgoers who never went to church as children, those adult non-churchgoers who went regularly as children show twice the level of Christian belief. In addition, the latter are more likely to hold moral attitudes on personal honesty and sexuality that are closer to those of regular churchgoers.

If this evidence is accurate it suggests, at least at an empirical level, that for many moral agents there is not the clear separation of morality and religion that the secular post-Enlightenment tradition has tended to claim. The latter may, at a more epistemological level, have underestimated the power of religious faith to motivate individual moral agents (or to use Fergusson's words cited earlier, 'the moral seriousness, commitment, and motivation which characterise a life of faith') and over-estimated its own power to resolve public

---

[31] Alasdair MacIntyre, *After Virtue: a Study in Moral Theory* (London: Duckworth, 2nd edn, 1985), pp. 268–9.

moral disagreements.[32] In contrast, in a world that is more self-consciously pluralistic, religious communities may once again be allowed a significant role in public debates about moral issues, even though they are unlikely to be granted the sort of monopoly of ethical decision-making more characteristic of theocracies than modern democracies.

Perhaps it is not surprising that public theology is now receiving increasing attention among academic theologians. On Duncan Forrester's retirement as director of the influential Centre for Theology and Public Issues at Edinburgh, twenty-four scholars from around the world contributed to the book *Public Theology for the 21st Century* to honour him. Raymond Plant depicted its publication as 'a very significant moment in the history of public theology over the past fifty or so years, taking stock of and renewing a sense of social vision in theology which we saw in earlier times exemplified in Gore and Temple and more recently in the work of Ronald Preston'.[33] Is it possible that public theology, in this sense, might even be able to redress the moral gaps that MacIntyre, Taylor and Hare have identified? This question needs to be addressed in the next chapter.

[32] For a well-informed evangelical analysis of this, see Scott B. Rae and Paul M. Cox (eds.), *Bioethics: a Christian Approach in a Pluralistic Age* (Grand Rapids, MI: William B. Eerdmans, 1999).

[33] Raymond Plant, 'Foreword', in William F. Storrar and Andrew R. Morton (eds.), *Public Theology for the 21st Century* (Edinburgh: T. & T. Clark, 2004), pp. x–xi.

CHAPTER 2

Tensions in public theology

The careful scholarship of Robin Lovin has done much to reveal a crucial tension at the heart of public theology. In his major study of Reinhold Niebuhr – whose influence as a public theologian in the mid-twentieth century was immense – he depicts the latter's position as follows:

Moral obligation is not meaningless apart from God. Specific moral obligations that transcend immediate interests can be defined without reference to divine commands or an ultimate center of value. Rather, God provides a reality in which a comprehensive unity of moral meanings is conceivable. It makes sense to seek genuine harmony between persons and groups, rather than to manage their conflicts prudently or to surrender to superior force, because human aspirations and values can be unified by the value they have in relationship to God. This unity both completes and transcends the partial resolutions of differences we anticipate in nature and history, and it impels those who apprehend it in faith to seek forms of justice that go beyond present expectations, even when that search involves considerable risk to themselves. The reality of God means that love, and not prudence, is the law of life.[1]

While Lovin seeks to defend this position, he is well aware that it is at odds with that dominant today in public theology. Increasingly it is now claimed by theologians that moral obligation really is 'meaningless apart from God'. They also tend to express considerable suspicion of other theologians who 'seek genuine harmony between persons and groups' outside explicit Christian faith.

In a review of recent Niebuhr scholarship, Lovin illustrates this tension by comparing the very different responses of Stanley

---

[1] Robin W. Lovin, *Reinhold Niebuhr and Christian Realism* (Cambridge and New York: Cambridge University Press, 1995), p. 67.

34

Hauerwas and Langdon Gilkey. Hauerwas argues at length that Niebuhr was finally a product of William James' pragmatism:

It appears that for Niebuhr God is nothing more than the name of our need to believe that life has an ultimate unity that transcends the world's chaos and makes possible what order we can achieve in this life. Niebuhr does not explain why he thinks anyone would feel compelled to worship or pray to a god so conceived.[2]

In complete contrast, Gilkey claims:

In Niebuhr's theology, God cannot be a projection, a human idea shone outward into the cosmos, an ideal, made transcendent by the creativity of human self-transcendence (though many of his statements in his early writings seemed to imply that view). Such a deity would for the mature Niebuhr be the creation of ordinary and all-too-common human idolatry, a product of a finite and so partial cultural imagination and so no more transcendent than any other cultural artefact.[3]

Understandably, Lovin concludes that 'their dramatically different readings of Niebuhr do suggest that more work remains to be done in interpreting his central ideas for our theological, cultural, and political situation today'.[4]

Tristram Engelhardt has relentlessly explored these tensions within Christian versions of health care ethics over the last decade. In the first issue of the journal that he was instrumental in establishing, *Christian Bioethics*, he wrote:

The Journal seeks to break new ground by taking the content of Christianity seriously while critically assessing the extent to which the different Christian faiths and their different health care policies authentically realize that content with respect to bioethical issues. Because Christians are separated, united neither in one communion nor in one baptism, *Christian Bioethics* will address differences, not just agreements ... It will seek to take seriously the commitments that divide Christians and which are appropriately bridged by conversion rather than by discounting differences.[5]

---

[2] Stanley Hauerwas, *With the Grain of the Universe: the Church's Witness and Natural Theology* (Grand Rapids, MI: Brazos Press, 2001), p. 131.

[3] Langdon Gilkey, *On Niebuhr: a Theological Study* (Chicago: University of Chicago Press, 2001), pp. 188–9.

[4] Robin W. Lovin, 'Reinhold Niebuhr in Contemporary Scholarship: a Review Essay', *Journal of Religious Ethics*, 31.3 (2003), p. 502.

[5] H. Tristram Engelhardt Jr, 'Towards a Christian Bioethics', *Christian Bioethics*, 1:1 (1995), pp. 1–2.

Engelhardt provocatively depicts this as a 'non-ecumenical' approach to Christian bioethics: an attempt to resist 'the temptations to make a Christian bioethics reach to all by conforming it to the generalities of a secular bioethics or an ecumenism of common commitments and roots'.[6] Even when he has invited contributors to address a common theme in the journal, he characteristically concludes by dwelling sharply on their internal differences. For example, in a more recent issue, he writes bluntly:

> This essay is implicitly critical of most of the contributors to this issue of *Christian Bioethics*. Most fail adequately to appreciate the moral and spiritual challenge to traditional Christian hospital chaplaincy. Once chaplaincy is defined by fully ecumenical professional norms, justifiable within the public discourse of a secular public space, chaplaincy takes on an identity independent of and hostile to traditional Christian concerns.[7]

How is the theological tension that so clearly divides Hauerwas, Engelhardt and Gilkey (and many other public theologians) to be depicted? And what implications does it have for those of us who are interested in exploring whether and how Christian ethics might still be able to make a significant contribution to health care ethics in the public forum of a Western, pluralistic society?[8]

COMPETING TYPOLOGIES

Academic theology is notoriously subject to swings of mood and temperament, with one dominant intellectual group being superseded by another as former students overturn the positions of those who taught them. In the twentieth century Karl Barth illustrated this process clearly. First he reacted sharply against the 'liberal' theologians of the pre-First World War period who taught him, then he attracted followers such as Dietrich Bonhoeffer in the crises leading up to the Second World War, then he was criticised by the so-called 'secular' theologians of the 1960s, and now he has become

---

[6] Engelhardt, 'Towards a Christian Bioethics', p. 6.

[7] H. Tristram Engelhardt Jr, 'The Dechristianization of Christian Hospital Chaplaincy: Some Bioethics Reflections on Professionalization, Ecumenization, and Secularization', *Christian Bioethics*, 9:1 (2003), p. 140.

[8] For a useful summary, see also Neil Messer (ed.), *Theological Issues in Bioethics* (London: DLT, 2002), ch. 10.

fashionable once more especially among younger theologians. The pendulum swings first to the left and then to the right and then to left and then ... Labels such as neo-orthodoxy, radical orthodoxy and critical theology are sometimes used to depict these different directions. Or sometimes it is the labels of traditionalism *versus* liberalism or even communitarianism *versus* liberalism. One way or another it at least is clear that academic theology is prone to swings of mood and temperament.

Viewed from the inside, theological controversies tend to appear as a straightforward battle between truth and error. That has typically been the stance of theological polemicists, whether they are Augustine in the fourth century, Luther in the sixteenth century or Barth in the twentieth century. For them theology is not a game, let alone some dispassionate academic exercise, but rather a battle for theological truth affecting the very survival of true Christian faith. Similarly theological controversies within Judaism or Islam have typically been about truth and error and, as a consequence, about the true identity of the Jewish or Islamic faith.

However, viewed sociologically, theological controversy is also about power, social reaction and generational shifts. The connection with power has long been evident in the *ex post facto* identification of theological orthodoxy by triumphant clerical elites. For example, in the controversies over infant baptism or the three-fold ministry (neither sanctioned explicitly within the New Testament) orthodoxy has been established by those who finally wrested power within a particular church. Indeed, on occasions clerical elites can even insist that a change in practice or belief away from long-established belief or practice represents orthodoxy – as happened, for example, with the swift introduction of the vernacular mass in the Roman Catholic Church. A connection between orthodoxy and power is well established among church historians and sociologists alike. (In passing it should of course be emphasised that from a theological perspective this connection does not actually invalidate the concept of orthodoxy, even though it might engender a certain amount of suspicion.)

A sociological perspective would also suggest a connection between theological controversy and both social reaction and generational shifts. To return to Barth, it is not difficult to suggest links between his sharp reaction against 'liberal' theological mentors so soon after the First World War both to the war itself and to his comparative youthfulness. Academic reputations are often established precisely by a younger generation showing where an older generation has been in error. In an accumulative discipline such as a science it is difficult for a younger generation to make a seismic shift away from the older generation (it takes a Darwin or an Einstein to do so convincingly). However, in many arts disciplines, especially where accumulative knowledge has less significance, such seismic generational shifts are commonplace. At the rather crude level of academic rivalry such shifts offer the young and ambitious ways of attempting to establish their academic reputations. At a more cognitive level, the very fact that many arts disciplines such as theology (or indeed sociology within the social sciences) have diametrically opposed methodologies and assumptions at their heart, always makes it possible for one generation to start in quite a different place or use a radically alternative methodology from the previous generation. Generational shifts in this non-science context are both tempting and easy.

What sociological ways of depicting and understanding these theological tensions and shifts are available? And which of these is finally the most useful? The word 'useful' here is important. An ideal typology within the sociology of religion is essentially a heuristic device, working best when it can generate insights and predictions both for sociologists and for the subjects of that typology. Sociologists of religion of an earlier generation (following Durkheim) were often quite content to produce typologies that ignored the self-understanding of the religious subjects that they studied. Today it is more common (following Weber) to include this self-understanding within the typology itself.

Among the typology options available are the following:
1. Orthodoxy *versus* heresy
2. Fundamentalism *versus* non-fundamentalism
3. Liberalism *versus* traditionalism
4. Liberalism *versus* conservatism
5. Liberalism/individualism *versus* communitarianism

The orthodoxy *versus* heresy typology falls at the first fence since few of those depicted as 'heretical' are likely to identify themselves with this label. And such an obvious product of theological polemics is also unlikely to commend itself to sociologists as a means of generating insights and predictions. An older generation of church historians, nurtured within particular ecclesiastical communities, might have regarded this typology as standard fare, but it would have fewer takers among their counterparts today.

The fundamentalism *versus* non-fundamentalism typology would appear to be just as vulnerable. It is clearly a distinction that is often made within theological polemics and those depicted as 'fundamentalists' are seldom happy with the label today. But there is a crucial difference here from the first typology. When first used by an American Baptist paper in 1920 it was adopted as a term of pride to depict 'those ready to do battle royal for the Fundamentals of Protestantism'.[9] The term was coined to depict those who could subscribe to a reassertion of biblical faith made in the twelve booklets *The Fundamentals* issued between 1910 and 1915 in order to counter critical biblical scholarship.[10] Some years ago in *Competing Convictions* I argued that these origins did provide a basis for depicting those who used scriptural absolutism (within Christianity, Judaism or Islam and perhaps even within Hinduism) to counter modernity. There I arrived at the following definition:

Fundamentalism may be tentatively defined as a system of beliefs and practices which treat scriptural absolutism as *the* way to counter the pluralism and relativism engendered by modernity. And the term militant fundamentalism might be used further to distinguish those recent forms of fundamentalism which have sought actively to counter modernity through political means.[11]

An important distinction needs to be observed here if the term 'fundamentalism' is to be used in this way. It would be anachronistic to depict earlier forms of scriptural absolutism, or even scriptural absolutism within present-day pre-modern societies, as 'fundamentalist'. *The Fundamentals* were a very specific reaction to critical biblical scholarship, so where the latter is unknown it cannot be depicted in this understanding as 'fundamentalist'.

---

[9] See E. Sandeen, *The Roots of Fundamentalism: British and American Millenarianism, 1800–1930* (Chicago: University of Chicago Press, 1970), p. 246.

[10] *The Fundamentals* (Chicago: Testimony Publishing Company, 1910–15).

[11] Robin Gill, *Competing Convictions* (London: SCM Press, 1989), p. 23.

With this distinction in mind it is quite tempting to apply the term 'fundamentalist' to those academic theologians who are currently employing scriptural or doctrinal absolutism to counter modernity. Theologians such as Stanley Hauerwas, John Milbank or Michael Banner regularly criticise the 'Enlightenment project' and refer disparagingly to 'liberal' theologians who are deemed to have bought into prevailing 'secular' assumptions. Each offers a distinctive set of theological absolutes that are then presented as a sharp counter to modernity. Although their books are manifestly more sophisticated than *The Fundamentals* it is arguable that their basic intentions are similar.

Yet the problem here is that not one of these theologians would be comfortable with a self-depiction as a 'fundamentalist'. The very term has too many crude overtones for this to be possible and manifestly (whatever its origins) it has now become a widespread term of abuse. Whether or not it can still be applied usefully within the global context of religious factions and political alliances, it would seem to present serious problems in depicting shifts within present-day academic theology.

The three other typologies all contain the term 'liberalism' and might be more useful. Hauerwas, Milbank and Banner do regularly depict themselves as opposed to 'liberals' and many of their theological adversaries might themselves be comfortable with this label. There is of course still some unease here. The political right under Ronald Reagan and Margaret Thatcher applied particular invective to the term 'liberal' ('the L word') and, among theologians at least, there is now often some hesitancy about using the term as a badge of honour. Nevertheless there is a case for arguing that there are enough self-styled liberal theologians and self-styled opponents of 'liberal theology' extant to make this a serious typological candidate.

Yet the problem about using the term 'liberal' in this context is to identify its opposite. If one group of theologians is to be depicted as 'liberal' just how are their theological opponents to be identified? There are at least three obvious candidates: traditionalists, conservatives, or communitarians. I suspect that the least popular self-depiction might be 'conservatives'. Exponents of Radical Orthodoxy such as John Milbank could scarcely be comfortable with the term 'conservative' and even the term 'traditionalist' may not feel too appropriate. Sociologists following Weber will also be aware that radical prophecy can be motivated either by a claim to new revelation or by an appeal to earlier tradition (or even by a mix of the two). The term 'traditionalist' is hardly without ambiguity.

A rather better case might be made for liberalism *versus* communitarianism. This does after all represent a tension to be found elsewhere in the academic world. On this understanding liberalism is almost synonymous with individualism. Undoubtedly there are some theologians who might be happy to be depicted as both liberals and individualists. Yet to depict all of the theological opponents of Hauerwas, Milbank and Banner in this way would be less than convincing. Besides, the specific academic debate between liberals and communitarians within philosophy and the social sciences is too recent to depict the generational shifts apparent within academic theology over the last century.

THEOLOGICAL PURITY *VERSUS* THEOLOGICAL REALISM

Uncomfortable with all five of these options, a sixth typology might be suggested based upon a distinction between theological purity and theological realism. Here theological purity is seen as a theological approach that seeks to derive doctrine and moral precepts exclusively from sacred texts and then to regard them as being in radical conflict with the secular world. In contrast, theological realism sees continuities between theological and secular thought and is sceptical about the capacity of sacred texts to deliver unambiguous doctrine let alone self-sufficient moral precepts in the modern world. The first of these positions tends to see a sharp contrast between the faithful and the secular world; it presupposes that the world at large is fundamentally secular, and that Christians (and, *mutatis mutandis*, Jews or Muslims) should look exclusively to their sacred texts (whether scriptural or patristic) to shape their beliefs and actions. The second, in contrast, does not make such a clear distinction between the faithful and the 'secular' world, tends to see the latter as more pluralist than secularist, and tends to regard sacred texts as key but not sufficient resources for belief and action today. Until recently Anglican theologians (William Temple and Ronald Preston are good examples) tended towards this second position. Within the United States, Reinhold Niebuhr and his heirs such as Robin Lovin provide obvious examples.

It might be hoped that neither side would be offended by such a self-depiction but could instead see it as a means to differentiate their own position from that of their theological opponents. At the heart of this typology is a real theological tension that confronts many religious traditions in the context of late modernity. Faithful religious adherents living in the religiously pluralist societies that characterise late modernity face this tension at many points in their lives. In premodern societies, characterised by comparative religious uniformity, this tension is either absent or much reduced. However, within late modernity the religiously faithful sometimes see an unattractive choice of living out their Christianity as 'a life-style option' or as 'resident aliens'.

It is important to remember that ideal typologies are indeed 'ideal' typologies: they are heuristic devices rather than straightforward empirical depictions. There are all sorts of options between theological purity and theological realism as depicted here. Further, an individual theologian may well appear in one mode as a theological purist and in another as a theological realist (Rowan Williams, and Michael Ramsey before him, are good examples of this, and, as a result, both tend to appeal to theological purists and theological realists alike). Instead, what this typology attempts to do is to depict a tension within theology in a context of late modernity and then to suggest that generational shifts among academic theologians can be seen as movements within this tension.

Seen in this way such generational shifts are also a reflection of the obvious point that neither side in this tension can realistically hope finally to triumph. It is not simply that the factors identified earlier (power, academic rivalry and the nature of non-accumulative academic disciplines) will militate against this. It is also that both sides of the tension between theological purists and theological realists have obvious weaknesses. The central weakness of theological purists is a tendency to claim too much and to fuel so-called 'culture wars'. It is after all unlikely that sacred texts will be able to deliver convincing verdicts on the perplexing array of moral dilemmas posed by late modernity, especially those dilemmas created by advances in recent physics, genetics or medicine. That is perhaps why theological purists often appear so anachronistic, and sometimes so divisive, in the public forum of a late-modern, pluralistic society. For some they may even appear dangerous. Writing himself as an African American theological realist, Preston Williams makes the telling point that 'the Christian failure in respect to racial justice made ... most African Americans aware of Christianity's imperfections in respect of truth ... Christianity was always seen as a mixture of culture, and religion, human talk and God's'.[12] The central weakness of theological realists is a tendency towards redundancy. By conceding too much to secular argument, theological realism always runs the risk of losing its identity altogether. As Lovin concedes, such theology 'is reduced to saying what everyone already believes' and, as a result, its inadequacy 'becomes more apparent over time, as beliefs change and what inspires one generation loses credibility with the next'.[13] If theological purity is prone to hyperbole, public irrelevance and divisive other-worldliness, theological realism is prone to evaporation and over-accommodating this-worldliness.

As Troeltsch foresaw in his classic study *The Social Teaching of the Christian Churches* (and F. D. Maurice, even earlier, in his *The Kingdom of Christ*), such a typology suggests an interesting point, relevant to both sociologists and to theologians. Having suggested a typology based upon tensions between churches, sects and individual mystics, Troeltsch then argued that together and in tension they represent Christianity in a fuller sense than they possibly could individually. So, despite the fact that each would like to eliminate the other, together they actually represent a greater whole. At a sociological level this is simply to acknowledge that a complex religious tradition contains tensions that constitute its very identity. However, at a theological level it suggests that Christianity (and again, *mutatis mutandis*, Judaism, Islam and perhaps many other religious traditions) is a sort of ecological ecumene. At an inter-religious theological level it might even suggest that apparently contradictory religious traditions could still constitute some form of

---

[12] Preston N. Williams, 'Christian Realism and the Ephesian Suggestion', *Journal of Religious Ethics*, 25:2 (1997), p. 238.
[13] Lovin, 'Niebuhr in Contemporary Scholarship', p. 499.

endlessly competing (and thus unharmonised ... this is not an argument for some perennial philosophy) ecological ecumene.

TWO EXAMPLES OF PUBLIC THEOLOGY

A broad examination of public theology would be inappropriate here. Instead, this chapter will focus upon a single question: what does theology have to contribute to public debates about ethical issues arising from recent genetic science? A number of scientists would respond emphatically that theology has nothing whatsoever to contribute. Even some religious scientists may be sceptical about any public role for theology on genetic issues. They may also be dismayed by what they regard as naïve theological utterances on specific scientific issues, especially on issues such as the genetic modification of food. In contrast, there is a growing theological literature relating to genetic and medical science which claims that a godless society is ever moving in a more destructive and irreligious direction, relegating powers to itself that properly belong only to God.

At a theological level there seems to be an increasing gap between those theologians who make sharply particularist claims (the theological purists) and those who see only relative differences between Christian and secular thought (the theological realists). Two books published in 1999 can be taken to illustrate this difference, Michael Banner's *Christian Ethics and Contemporary Moral Problems*[14] and Audrey R. Chapman's *Unprecedented Choices: Religious Ethics at the Frontiers of Genetic Science.*[15] Since both Michael Banner and Audrey Chapman are themselves involved as theologians on public bodies concerned with genetics and health care ethics, their work is directly relevant to this question about public theology. In theory, at least, they represent opposite positions on public theology, with Banner an enthusiastic Barthian and particularist, the theological purist, and Chapman as more consensual and sympathetic to process theology, the theological realist. In practice, as will be seen, their differences are

---

[14] Michael Banner, *Christian Ethics and Contemporary Moral Problems* (Cambridge: Cambridge University Press, 1999).

[15] Audrey R. Chapman, *Unprecedented Choices: Religious Ethics at the Frontiers of Genetic Science* (Minneapolis: Fortress Press, 1999).

not so clear-cut. This final observation will lead to a summary of my own position, namely that religious beliefs are important for critical depth and parameters, as well as for motivation, on ethical issues even in a pluralistic society. It is when public theologians imagine that, by virtue of being theologians, they have some all-encompassing capacity for moral discernment on complex issues in genetic and medical science that they can be most misleading. To save them from error they need their secular colleagues. Conversely secular colleagues may sometimes underestimate the critical depth, parameters and motivation which religious belonging and beliefs (or the heritage deriving from them) can still give people when making difficult ethical choices.

AUDREY CHAPMAN

Audrey Chapman's *Unprecedented Choices: Religious Ethics at the Frontiers of Genetic Science* sets out to provide an informed critical discussion of both the implications of recent genetic science for religious ethics and the contribution that religious ethics have made, or might still make, for society at large as it attempts to evaluate the ethical and social implications of this science. As director of the Program of Dialogue on Science, Ethics and Religion at the American Association for the Advancement of Science at Washington, DC, she has a decade of active engagement with religious leaders, theologians and scientists on genetic issues, attempting to establish properly informed and credible responses. However this has left her less than sanguine about the contribution to date of religious ethicists on the crucial issues increasingly raised by genetic science.

Three substantial chapters survey, in turn, the contributions of religious ethicists first to the possibility of human genetic engineering, then to the possibility of human cloning and finally to the ongoing debate about the patenting of life. Those who have been engaged actively in the current debate will be very familiar with the issues and arguments used and Chapman adds little that is new in the first and second of these areas. Nonetheless, what she does write is clear, accurate and perceptive. Because she adopts a survey style in these chapters, rather than a thematic approach, there is a considerable amount of repetition of points, arguments and even quotations. She is also not particularly aware of parallel British and European discussions. As in the United States, a number of British religious ethicists have been discussing genetic issues over the last decade and most British Government or Foundation reports on genetics and ethics have included religious ethicists in their panels. An adequate survey should include more of these non-American contributions, although it would probably not add much to the actual substance of the debate. There are as yet only so many points to be made about the merits or otherwise of novel but circumscribed areas such as genetic engineering or reproductive cloning.

It is in the third area – on the patenting of life – that Chapman makes a distinctly more original contribution. She takes as her starting point the 'Joint Appeal Against Human and Animal Patenting' made in May 1995 by more than eighty religious leaders. The 'Joint Appeal' opposed the patenting of human and animal life forms on the following grounds:

We the undersigned religious leaders, oppose the patenting of human and animal life forms. We are disturbed by the US Patent Office's recent decision to patent human body parts and several genetically engineered animals. We believe that humans and animals are creations of God, not humans, and as such should not be patented as human inventions.[16]

Instructively this is the area that has most actively concerned her work for the American Association for the Advancement of Science. Because of the legal complications in this area, debate about it has been particularly convoluted both in the United States and in Europe. Chapman offers a useful guide through this legal minefield and a clarification of the specifically ethical issues identified in the secular debate, before turning at some length to the theological issues involved. It is at this point that she offers her critique of what she sees as the simplicities of the 'Joint Appeal'. She argues that there has been a long-standing tendency of religious leaders in such debates to offer rhetoric rather than properly informed argument. For example, as it stands, she believes that the 'Joint Appeal' depends upon a static, pre-evolutionary understanding of creation in

---

[16] General Board of Church and Society of the United Methodist Church, 'Joint Appeal Against Human and Animal Patenting' (press conference announcement), Washington, DC, 17 May 1995.

which life-forms are firmly fixed by God. It also has an unnuanced understanding of 'ownership' that takes no account of the concept of humans as 'created co-creators' developed by the theologians Philip Hefner and Ted Peters. She is also sceptical about the legitimacy of religious leaders speaking on behalf of their faith traditions without extensive prior consultation of a strong cross-section of their members.

However, Chapman still believes in public theology and in religious ethicists seeking to influence society at large, especially on ethical issues. The two chapters that follow offer an extensive discussion first of how theologians should take more account of scientific developments and then of how they should seek to engage in public theology. At the first of these levels she believes that most theologians have still to assimilate the implications of Darwin and modern genetics properly into their understanding of creation, human distinctiveness, sin and the soul. She examines the claims of sociobiology and, like Stephen Pope, is sympathetic to a judicious assimilation even here (although she is also critical of some of the more exaggerated claims of sociobiologists such as Richard Dawkins and Edward O. Wilson). At the second level she argues repeatedly that public theology in the area of genetic science should succumb neither to the abandonment of theistic language (she is particularly critical of James Childress for failing to make his theological premises apparent in *Principles of Biomedical Ethics*) nor to simplistic biblical or theological claims.

This last point is crucial to all of us who work as religious ethicists alongside physical and social scientists. What is the responsible way to do religious ethics on scientific issues within pluralistic, modern societies? Chapman is well aware that some secular scientists would exclude religious ethicists from any discussion that impinges upon their work. She counters this with the position taken by the National Bioethics Advisory Commission, namely that the claims of religious traditions should be taken seriously, without being regarded as determinative, because historically and currently they mould the moral views of many citizens. Once it is acknowledged that secularists themselves do not arrive at moral positions independently of culture, then there is a strong ground for not excluding any significant section of a particular culture.

An additional point might be made here to strengthen this position. It is sometimes argued that, although neither religious bodies nor their theologians can properly claim to represent society as a whole today (in the USA, of course, they never could, but at times both the Church of England and the Church of Scotland, have imagined that, in England and Scotland at least, they can), secular moral philosophy might be able to make such a claim in a pluralistic society. It was, as argued in the previous chapter, one of the central hopes of the Enlightenment that the use of universal reason without the particularist claims of divine revelation might help to deliver Europe from inter-religious wars. European countries fractured by the Protestant Reformation could no longer unanimously rely upon religiously derived moral precepts. Morality based solely upon universal human reasoning might instead be able to unite people morally in a way that religion no longer could. However, as already argued, the 'moral gaps' in secular health care ethics make such a position distinctly less plausible. And, in any case, rivalries between different theoretical positions in moral philosophy are just as evident as those among theologians.

So, in a discussion of the public role of applied ethics, my colleague, the secular philosopher Richard Norman, has argued that 'if the resolution of moral conflicts about abortion, or euthanasia, has to wait the resolution of disputes between utilitarianism, rights-based theories, and their other theoretical competitors, there is little hope of progress towards agreed answers'.[17] Instead, Norman argues more modestly that the function of the philosopher in public ethical decision-making is be concerned with 'the clarification and articulation of the values which people actually hold'.[18] Rather than insisting upon some unified theory or set of principles, philosophy in this area 'consists in the attempt to understand and clarify, non-reductively, the plurality of ethical values and concepts'.[19]

Given such a modest understanding of the role of secular philosophy in the public forum, it is not so difficult to imagine that the theologian may have some public role as well. Yet it is at this point

[17] Richard Norman, 'Applied Ethics: What is Applied to What?', *Utilitas*, 12:2 (July 2000), p. 131.
[18] Norman, 'Applied Ethics', p. 131.   [19] Norman, 'Applied Ethics', p. 136.

that Chapman's own position becomes more problematic. Her book is strongest when exposing the inadequacies of various religious positions, either because they fail properly to understand genetic science or because they make tendentious connections between theology and particular claims or prescriptions relating to genetic science. Such versions of public theology thus fail either at the cognitive or at the hermeneutical level. Yet her own positive connections are quite tentative and are seldom distinctively theological. So, although she argues that genetic patenting does raise important theological questions, she leaves these questions articulated rather than answered. And when looking for something positive to say about the 'Joint Appeal' she writes only in general (and non-theological) terms:

Like the members of the Joint Appeal campaign, I am disturbed by the failure to have a meaningful public discussion of this issue. The courts and the patenting office are not the proper venue for making such decisions. To embark on a course of promoting commercialisation and privatisation of biology without a single meaningful public debate constitutes a violation of the implicit social contract between the government and the governed in a democratic society.[20]

And when she does address directly how it is that religious ethicists tend to differ from secular ethicists, she points to three distinct ways: religious ethicists are more likely than secular ethicists to move beyond individual autonomy and consent and to emphasise wider interpersonal and social relationships; they are more committed to justice and concern for the vulnerable; and they belong to religious communities with uniquely long traditions of moral discussion and attention to moral behaviour.

It can indeed be agreed that all three are both distinct and crucial to the role of a number of theologians who work with secular bodies. Yet all of these are derivative virtues rather than the explicitly doctrinal claims usually advanced by purist exponents of public theology. What is more, such differences between religious and secular ethicists are, at most, relative differences. Manifestly there are secular ethicists (for example, secular communitarians) who are deeply

[20] Chapman, *Unprecedented Choices*, p. 162.

concerned about wider interpersonal relationships and about justice for the vulnerable, as well as secular ethicists who value long traditions of moral discussion (moral philosophy itself can claim a lengthy history). There are also some religious ethicists who are distinctly individualistic in style and dismissive of religious traditions on moral issues. All that can be safely claimed here is that religious ethicists in general are more likely than their secular counterparts to enshrine these three derivative virtues. At most this is a relative rather than substantive difference between religious and secular ethicists.

But what about distinctive theologically based arguments in public theology? Chapman claims briefly that there is a greater tolerance in secular society today for such arguments (but, tellingly, she makes this claim for theistic rather than Christological arguments). Perhaps this is true in the United States as a whole (although it is doubtful if it is true in the secular academy in the US), but it is not the case in Britain or more widely in much of Europe. Memories of religious wars and/or religious hegemonies in the latter are still too recent for this to be possible. Given this, the religious ethicist engaged in the genetics debate within the public forum may simply have to chose: either to use explicitly religious arguments and, in the process, inform their religious communities but be ignored largely by society at large; or to represent the virtues of social concern and justice derived from their communities while largely eschewing public discussion of theological meta-ethics. Those from the first position often regard those from the second as faithless, whereas those from the second tend to regard those from the first as sectarian. Neither label withstands much intelligent scrutiny[21] since these differing positions are as much public strategies as ontologies. Yet they remain difficult to resolve and continue to have a profound affect upon religious ethics at the frontiers of genetic research.

MICHAEL BANNER

In 1993 Michael Banner was appointed to chair a government committee on farm animals, which produced *The Report of the Committee*

---

[21] See David Fergusson, *Community, Liberalism and Christian Ethics* (Cambridge: Cambridge University Press, 1998).

to Consider the Ethical Implications of Emerging Technologies in the Breeding of Farm Animals,[22] then to the F. D. Maurice Chair of Moral and Social Theology at King's College London and more recently to the Chair of Public Policy in the Life Sciences at Edinburgh University. In 1999 he published his first substantial collection of essays on ethical issues, *Christian Ethics and Contemporary Moral Problems*. It offers a sharp contrast to Chapman. In the opening chapter of this book, his inaugural lecture at King's, he argues for a particularist theological approach to Christian ethics, which he terms 'dogmatic Christian ethics'. He argues that the only authorities for Christian ethics are the Bible and the Creeds – although, in reality, it is Karl Barth whom he treats as the authority in almost every chapter that follows. In these he considers, in turn, euthanasia, abortion, health care rationing, the environment, biotechnology and sexuality – concluding, provocatively, with a 'prolegomena to a dogmatic sexual ethic'. Throughout he makes his mark as a radical theological purist:

Where Christian ethics understands itself as dogmatic ethics – that is, as providing an account of human action as it corresponds to the reality of the action of God – it necessarily understands itself in such a way as to differentiate itself from a number of other accounts of ethics, even when those are given from the Christian side.[23]

He is highly critical of those forms of public theology which seek to find common ground between religious and secular ethicists and argues that a sharply particularist approach to Christian ethics offers a more significant dialogue partner even within a pluralist society. In turn this leads him to defend such an approach within health care ethics:

Christian medical ethics, in so far as it is *Christian* medical ethics, speaks on the basis of the distinctive knowledge of humankind which is given by the Word of God. It thus does not and cannot make common cause with 'bioethics', or 'biomedical ethics', as they are usually practised, for as thus practised they do not view humankind in the light of this knowledge. Christian medical ethics is, rather, obliged to begin from its own starting point, taking up the constructive task from its unique and distinctive

---

[22] London: HMO, 1995.   [23] Banner, *Christian Ethics*, p. 13.

presupposition, namely the Gospel of Jesus Christ. For it is in the light of this Gospel of the Word spoken to humankind, that humankind gains a true self-understanding.[24]

Banner's sharp-edged theological purity makes him an effective critic of sloppy, 'realist' writing. Secular exponents of consequentialism in moral philosophy are dissected with considerable panache. Aware that in a pluralist context it becomes ever more difficult to argue for agreed moral principles of any kind, he fears that there is a real danger that measurable consequence will become the only public guide on moral issues. He successfully shows just how impoverished a stance that would be. Yet, on issues such as abortion, euthanasia and homosexuality, which he implacably opposes, he comes near to arguing that consequences should simply be ignored. Even if prudence is not all, principles alone (so it will be argued in chapter 4) can be less than compassionate.

However, it is striking that, when he comes to the area of ethics in which he has a public role himself (namely on the environment and farm animals), he allows prudence a much greater place and eschews 'black and white' solutions. He criticises other genetic reports for being purely consequentialist – when in reality they typically combine consequentialism and deontology – while offering a mixture of consequentialism and deontology himself – a mixture that then sits uneasily with the dogmatic Christian ethics with which he concludes. For example, he cites the following paragraph from the BMA report *Our Genetic Future* as typifying secular consequentialism:

Using the science of genetic modification to produce a 'master race', or to select children with particular attributes, is unacceptable. Even if parents are entirely free to reproduce as they choose, considerable social and ethical problems could arise if we eventually reach the currently remote possibility of being able to choose not just the gender but also some of the physical, emotional, and intellectual attributes of our children. If it became commonplace, for example, for parents to choose a boy as their first child, then this might well make it even harder to diminish sexual discrimination in our society.[25]

[24] Banner, *Christian Ethics*, pp. 48–9.
[25] British Medical Association, *Our Genetic Future: the Science and Ethics of Genetic Technology* (Oxford: Oxford University Press, 1992), p. 209.

Clearly consequentialism is present in this argument, but 'sexual discrimination' seems to be regarded deontologically as simply wrong in itself. And the conditional clause at the beginning of the second sentence suggests that parental autonomy may not be decisive here. A careful reading of the rest of the report and almost any other report of the BMA Medical Ethics Committee would soon confirm that the deontological principles of justice and non-maleficence are regularly considered alongside autonomy and beneficence. What Banner tries to show is that other reports on issues in genetics rely exclusively upon a consequentialist balance between 'risks' and 'benefits' and thereby overlook the possibility that some things may be wrong in themselves. Perhaps some do, but it is difficult to find evidence of this in the sophisticated reports produced by bodies such as the BMA or the Nuffield Council on Bioethics. And even the term 'benefits' allows for other possibilities.

When in the 1980s I first started discussions with scientists involved in biotechnology I found that some talked simply about risk analysis without any mention of beneficence. At that stage such scientists were puzzled about why ethics (let alone theology) had anything to do with their work at all. However, once it is acknowledged that biotechnology should be as concerned about whether or not it really does contribute towards beneficence, the role of the ethicist becomes more obvious to the scientists themselves. Clearly this in itself raises the issues of what constitutes 'beneficence' and whether it is right that some should benefit at the risk of possible harm to other people, to animals or to the environment. Thoroughgoing consequentialists can doubtless avoid deontological principles even when addressing these issues, but they have to be unusually determined to do so. Most people (whether religious or not) offer a mixture of consequentialism and deontology in moral arguments.

And that is exactly what Michael Banner does himself. He cites with approval the three principles which his own report enunciates, namely a deontological principle that there are harms of a certain degree and kind which ought never to be inflicted upon animals (such as the non-therapeutic tongue amputation of calves), a more consequentialist principle that even less serious harm to animals must be weighed against the good to be achieved, and a third deontological principle that harm to animals should always be minimised. He also argues against a deontological position that seeks to prevent all forms of genetic engineering on animals, arguing as follows:

> If things were black and white it would, of course, be a lot easier. If the effect of genetic engineering were invariably deleterious for an animal's welfare, or if the very use of genetic modifications expressed a contempt for animals and a disregard for their natural characteristics (as some objections to genetic engineering maintain) a system of regulation might be devised which would aim to prevent all genetic modification . . . As it is, however, genetic modification cannot be regarded as a single moral entity – some genetic modification may be intrinsically objectionable as manipulative of an animal's good, some not.[26]

The Christian philosopher and radical vegetarian Stephen Clark would take a much more robust position here, rejecting all such genetic modification on deontological grounds.[27] In contrast to his univocal moral stances against abortion, euthanasia and homosexual practice, Banner is more cautious on this public issue.

Yet when he turns to theology in the conclusion of this discussion he appears to reject genetic engineering altogether and suspects that those Christians who talk about humans acting as 'co-creators' may 'serve only to provide to projects which may repudiate rather than embrace the created order an air of pious respectability'.[28] He also returns to his attack upon consequentialism:

> For what this line of questioning wonders is not just whether projects, for example, of perfective (as opposed to therapeutic) genetic engineering will have a balance of good over bad consequences, but rather whether they express a fundamentally mistaken attitude towards human being in the world, an attitude which will be overcome only as we learn what it means to keep the Sabbath as a day on which humankind is called to a knowledge and love of the order which God himself knows and loves.[29]

Now of course this last theological consideration could be an argument against any scientific intervention within 'the order which God himself knows and loves'. On this basis some

---

[26] Banner, *Christian Ethics*, pp. 218–19.
[27] See Stephen R. L. Clark, *Biology and Christian Ethics* (Cambridge: Cambridge University Press, 2000).
[28] Banner, *Christian Ethics*, p. 224.   [29] Banner, *Christian Ethics*, p. 224.

Christians have concluded that we must reject the whole of modern medicine and others that we must become thoroughgoing vegans. Yet most Christians, including Michael Banner, have not adopted such absolutist positions. For us theological considerations about God's creation have not univocally resolved our ethical dilemmas about biotechnology.[30]

So both Banner and Chapman, despite approaching genetic science from very different theological perspectives, appear to reach a very similar point. On other moral issues (in which, instructively, he is not so engaged in the public forum) Banner's position is typically absolutist and particularist, but on genetics (on which he is publicly engaged) he, like Chapman, generally eschews 'black and white' solutions.

THE ROLE OF PUBLIC THEOLOGY IN HEALTH CARE ETHICS

So perhaps the moral to be drawn from these two examples of public theology is simply that theologians should not be engaged at all in such a public forum in a late-modern, pluralistic society. Because, if they do get so engaged, they inevitably compromise their theological convictions. Better to live as Christians within our distinctive communities but apart from the public forum than to be compromised and relativised by the latter. Under the huge influence of Stanley Hauerwas within Christian ethics, quite a number of theologians today appear to be adopting this stance. More than anyone else Hauerwas has challenged theologians to think more carefully about the distinctively Christian resources that we bring to ethical issues and to take virtue ethics seriously. He has also raised doubts about those of us who still regard these resources as being compatible with more secular forms of ethics in the public forum.

Hauerwas can be at his most persuasive when writing about health care ethics, for example in his profound book *Suffering Presence*[31] or in *Naming the Silences*.[32] He requires readers to think about issues

---

[30] For similar theological criticism of the position that Banner respresents, see Celia Deane-Drumond, *Genetics and Christian Ethics* (Cambridge: Cambridge University Press, 2005).

[31] Stanley Hauerwas, *Suffering Presence* (Notre Dame, IN and Edinburgh: University of Notre Dame Press, 1986 and T. & T. Clark, 1988).

[32] Stanley Hauerwas, *Naming the Silences* (Grand Rapids, MI: William B. Eerdmans, 1990).

such as mental health care in ecclesial rather than secular terms. The method he proposes arises from the convictions about the vital connection he made in the early 1980s between virtue ethics and the church as a distinctive community:

any consideration of the truth of Christian convictions cannot be divorced from the kind of community the church is and should be ... my primary interest is to challenge the church to regain a sense of the significance of the polity that derives from convictions peculiar to Christians ... if the church is to serve our liberal society or any society, it is crucial for Christians to regain an appropriate sense of separateness from that society.[33]

Later in the same book he also wrote:

The contention and witness of the church is that the story of Jesus provides a flourishing of gifts which other politics cannot know. It does so because Christians have been nourished on the story of a savior who insisted on being nothing else than what he was. By being the son of God he provided us with the confidence that insofar as we become his disciples our particularity and our regard for the particularity of our brothers and sisters in Christ contribute to his Kingdom. Our stories become part of the story of the Kingdom.[34]

Although I have been critical elsewhere[35] of Hauerwas' emphasis upon the 'separateness' and even 'alienation' of the church from secular society that has increasingly dominated his recent writings, I still believe in an ecclesial Christian virtue ethic centred upon the story of Jesus. Where I differ from him in ecclesial terms is in my belief that such an ethic can complement, deepen and sometimes challenge, but not simply replace (except of course in gross circumstances such as the Nazi medical 'experiments' upon prisoners), a purely secular account of health care ethics. Where I differ theologically is in my growing conviction that the primary biblical resource for such an ethic is to be located in the Synoptic healing stories rather than in the Pauline corpus. The next chapter will attempt to take this

[33] Stanley Hauerwas, *A Community of Character: Toward a Constructive Christian Social Ethic* (Notre Dame, IN: University of Notre Dame Press, 1981), pp. 1–2.

[34] Hauerwas, *A Community of Character*, p. 51.

[35] See Robin Gill, *Churchgoing and Christian Ethics* (Cambridge: Cambridge University Press, 1999), ch. 3. See also Stephen E. Lammers, 'On Stanley Hauerwas: Theology, Medical Ethics, and the Church', in Allen Verhey and Stephen E. Lammers (eds.), *Theological Voices in Medical Ethics* (Grand Rapids, MI: William B. Eerdmans, 1993), pp. 74–6.

theological conviction a stage further by looking carefully at the explicit or implicit virtues contained in these Synoptic healing stories as a primary resource for health care ethics today.

Identifying implicit assumptions, beliefs and practices – sometimes at odds with those that are explicitly stated – is germane to social science. Both quantitative and qualitative methods can be used to achieve this in the modern world, as I attempted to demonstrate at length in *Churchgoing and Christian Ethics*. In the ancient world it is likely to be qualitative methods alone that are appropriate. However, by using such methods effectively, it might be possible to analyse the healing stories in the Synoptic Gospels to uncover the virtues implicit within them.

The position that I will seek to explore is that such theological considerations can bring critical depth and parameters, as well as moral motivation, to health care ethics and even to genetic issues. However, moral discernment in the complex and fast-changing world of genetic science (and, indeed, innovations in health care more widely) is possible only if theologians are prepared to listen carefully to their colleagues in science and moral philosophy. On complex ethical issues arising from genetic and medical science, neither theology nor church bodies have privileged access to moral discernment.

The philosopher William Frankena adopts a similar, realist position, arguing that theological presuppositions do provide both a rationality and motivation for ethical enquiry but cannot in themselves resolve problems of interpretation and application in such complex and novel areas as biotechnology.[36] Having worked directly alongside Richard Norman, I have learned to respect his role as a philosopher attempting 'to understand and clarify, non-reductively, the plurality of ethical values and concepts'. Even if theologians are suspicious at times of the depth, critical parameters or motivation of some of their secular colleagues, they have no privileged access to moral discernment on issues such as those raised by genetic science.

Within the New Studies in Christian Ethics series, the contributions that are closest to my own theological realist position are those of David Fergusson, Robert Gascoigne and Douglas Hicks.

---

[36] W. K. Frankena, 'The Potential of Theology for Ethics', in E. E. Shelp (ed.), *Theology and Bioethics* (Dordrecht: D. Reidel, 1985), pp. 49–64.

As already noted in the previous chapter, Fergusson criticises MacIntyre for not taking sufficient note of 'the moral seriousness, commitment, and motivation which characterise a life of faith'.[37] However, in the opposite direction, he is just as concerned about Hauerwas' 'principal weakness', namely, an 'overdetermination of the distinctiveness of the church ... an attenuated reading of the person and work of Christ, and ... a reluctance to describe the possibility of ethical perception and action outwith the Christian community'.[38] In short, this is the central weakness of a position in public theology based solely upon theological purity.

From an explicitly Catholic position, Robert Gascoigne also resists the thoroughgoing purist position that Hauerwas adopts. Hauerwas, he argues, has an 'emphasis on the need for Christians to confront the stark differences between the praxis of Jesus and the ways of this world, and to hear his words as an inspiration to a form of discipleship that radically negates the forces and interests that dominate society'.[39] Gascoigne, in contrast, favours the theological realism typified by Rahner:

For Karl Rahner, the Christian Gospel is the final and definitive form of humanity's historical attempt to give categorical or explicit shape to its experience of transcendental revelation, of the grace of God. The universal intention of the Gospel gives us grounds for interpreting and illuminating all of human existence in its light. All human religion, however primitive and distorted, is a response to that experience of the self-communication of God which constitutes our specifically human creatureliness. It is the Gospel, and only the Gospel, which enables us to interpret human existence in this way – without it we would have no ultimate assurance of the nearness and friendliness of God. Yet, in the light of the Gospel, we can reflect on the ways in which other religions and philosophies express aspects of ultimate truth.[40]

Gascoigne also argues at length against the theological purity of John Milbank:

For Milbank, Rahner's mistake was to begin from the universal human experience, and to seek to add a Christian dimension to this. Milbank

---

[37] Fergusson, *Community*, p. 136.   [38] Fergusson, *Community*, p. 67.

[39] Robert Gascoigne, *The Public Forum and Christian Ethics* (Cambridge: Cambridge University Press, 2001), p. 99.

[40] Gascoigne, *Public Forum*, p. 100.

argues that this implies that we have access to such experience in a way that is independent of narrative. Further, it implies an acceptance of the validity of 'secular reason' in interpreting this experience, and of the validity of a dialogue between Christian faith and 'secular reason' in achieving a full understanding of the relationship between sacred and secular. None of this is compatible with Milbank's own view that Christianity and 'secular reason' are competing 'total interpretations' of reality.[41]

Such a position clearly offends Gascoigne's more typically Catholic theological position. He insists that 'for Rahner, transcendence and historicity are not opposed but, rather, complementary: the human person develops and expresses transcendent freedom through involvement in historical situations'. And this he sees as a legitimate 'attempt to understand the transcendence of the human person *in the light* of Christian faith, in a way which allows contemporary human beings to explore the relationships and analogies between their own experience and the Christian tradition'.[42]

Douglas Hicks' contribution to New Studies in Christian Ethics adopts a similar theological realist position in his extended analysis of inequality.[43] His primary inspiration (as indicated already in the Introduction) is the secular economist Amartya Sen's notion of 'equality of basic capability'. Hicks argues that Christian ethics can contribute at three distinctive levels: by providing a moral vision and justification for how inequality matters and why public response is needed; by offering moral examples of Christians who have actively striven against inequality; and by providing a particularly compelling moral call to action. I suspect that both Hauerwas and Milbank would vigorously resist such a project and see it simply as capitulation to 'secular reason'. While stimulated by their robust challenge, my own project is finally much nearer to that of Hicks.

To return to Chapman and Banner, both hold that Christian ethics still has a distinctive critical function within the public

---

[41] Gascoigne, *Public Forum*, pp. 144–5.

[42] Gascoigne, *Public Forum*, pp. 150–1. For similar Catholic critiques of Milbank, see Aidan Nichols, 'Non Tali Auxilio: John Milbank's Suasion to Orthodoxy', *New Blackfriars*, 73:861 (1992), pp. 326–32, and John Orme Mills' new Introduction to the reprinted David Martin, John Orme Mills and W. S. F. Pickering (eds.), *Sociology and Theology: Alliance and Conflict* (Leiden and Boston: Brill, 2004), p. 12.

[43] Douglas A. Hicks, *Inequality and Christian Ethics* (Cambridge: Cambridge University Press, 2000).

forum. Whether this takes the form of questioning the sufficiency of autonomy as a moral principle or of pointing towards justice and concern for the vulnerable (Chapman), or whether it entails reminding a pluralist society of the theological roots of many assumed values (Banner), there does seem to be a critical public role for the theologian. Elsewhere[44] I have argued that public theology has a threefold critical role – criticising, deepening and widening the ethical debate in society at large. The deepening and widening aspects depend upon theistic and christological assumptions, offering a vision for those who will hear of how things could be if all shared these assumptions and were committed to a Christian *eschaton*. Where my position differs from both Chapman and Banner is in expecting that the second and third functions can play a role in the direct work of public bodies concerned with ethics. The latter should remain sensitive to the beliefs of those who are religious within society at large, but it would be inappropriate in a pluralist context for them to adopt explicit theological beliefs themselves. Indeed, public bodies are likely to regard such explicit adoption not just as inappropriate but, given their fear of religious wars, as dangerously partisan.

On occasions it is the role of a theologian on such bodies to remind them of a need for sensitivity towards religious minorities. Yet, ironically, it is as likely to be sensitivity towards the beliefs of Jehovah's Witnesses as towards those of mainstream practising Christians or Jews. More often the role is the incremental one that Lovin accurately portrays:

In a complex world where moral purposes are implemented by morally ambiguous institutions and powers, a form of ethics that understands those institutions and powers and speaks to them in their own terms seems best suited to the task of achieving what justice can do . . . The practical task of moral leadership is to convince those who think the achievement is too small to bother with that 'a little more justice' is still important, and to convince those who think they can do more that 'a little more justice' as a real achievement is better than a whole new order of good intentions.[45]

---

[44] See Robin Gill, *Moral Leadership in a Postmodern Age* (Edinburgh: T. & T. Clark, 1997), pp. 6f.
[45] Lovin, 'Niehbuhr in Contemporary Scholarship', p. 490.

And finally there is the role of religious commitment (described at the end of the previous chapter) as an important source of ethical motivation for individuals and for religious activism. Intellectual theologians and secular ethicists alike are apt to overlook this. Yet there is now considerable empirical evidence showing that religious belonging and stated moral attitudes and behaviour are closely connected. These connections are never absolute. Values and patterns of moral behaviour are distributed throughout the population, but some, especially those concerned with altruism and moral order, are clustered among those who are explicitly religious. And, as Lisa Cahill correctly argues, they are crucial to religious activism. Richard Norman does not discuss this, but his formulation of applied ethics does allow for it. He does not suggest that it is the function of the philosopher to inspire or engender moral values but rather to understand and clarify 'the values which people actually hold'. Presumably this includes both the values that explicitly religious people hold as well as the religiously derived values of those who are not or are no longer explicitly religious themselves. Indeed, there is growing empirical evidence (to be reviewed further in chapter 6), suggesting that religious belonging and motivation has often been underestimated in health care. Religious factors may yet be more significant in the public realm than is often realised. While seeking to avoid pontificating beyond their own data, public theologians could – so it will be argued later – make fuller use of this intriguing evidence.

CHAPTER 3

Healing in the Synoptic Gospels

The most obvious and most abundant theological resource on healing is the stories in the Synoptic Gospels. Mark's Gospel alone contains thirteen healing stories (most with parallels in Matthew and/or Luke) together with four general summaries of healings. There are also two further healing stories contained in the joint material in Matthew and Luke, five in Luke alone and three in Matthew alone. Healing stories are also recounted in John and Acts, but they are less frequent.

Given the sheer abundance of the Synoptic healing stories there can be little doubt that, whatever the difficulties there are in establishing other incontestable data about the historical ministry of Jesus, it was much concerned with healing. There is a rare point of agreement here among recent biblical scholars. To give just three examples, Howard Clark Kee, Gerd Theissen and Bruce J. Malina – all scholars who have made a major contribution to understanding the social world of the New Testament – agree that the Synoptic healing stories really do reflect Jesus' historical ministry.

Howard Clark Kee concludes in his *Medicine, Miracle and Magic in New Testament Times*:

The phenomenon of healing in the gospels and elsewhere in the New Testament is a central factor in primitive Christianity, and was so from the beginning of the movement. It is not a later addendum to the tradition, introduced in order to make Jesus more appealing to the Hellenistic world, but was a major feature of the Jesus tradition from the outset. Indeed, it is almost certainly a part of the historical core of that tradition, even though it is likely to have been embellished in the process of transmission. The performance of miracles in first-century Judaism is adequately attested even though the significance given to it in the Jesus tradition – signs of the inbreaking of the New Age – is a distinctive development of the apocalyptic tradition, especially as we see it in Daniel. As the gospels attest, and as the evidence of the Hellenistic healing cults suggests, the performance of healings and exorcisms by Jesus was seen as a central factor in the rapidly developed movement that Jesus called forth in Palestine and Syria, as well as in the astonishing spread of Christianity throughout the Mediterranean world.[1]

In his major work *The Miracle Stories of the Early Christian Tradition* Gerd Theissen also sees healing stories, and miracles more generally, as being of central importance both to Jesus and to earliest Christianity. He, too, insists, that:

There is no doubt that Jesus worked miracles, healed the sick and cast out demons, but the miracle stories reproduce these historical events in an intensified form. However, this enhancement of the historical and factual begins with Jesus himself. For Jesus too the miracles were not normal events, but elements in a mythical drama: in them the miraculous transformation of the world into [the Kingdom of God] was being carried out. As an apocalyptic charismatic miracle-worker, Jesus is unique in religious history. He combines two conceptual worlds which had never been combined in this way before, the apocalyptic expectation of universal salvation in the future and the episodic realisation of salvation in the present through miracles.[2]

Nor is Theissen impressed with earlier scholars who used redaction criticism to reduce the importance of miracles in the early church. In his view 'the alleged reservations of New Testament redactors about the miracles turn out on closer examination to be almost always reservations by modern exegetes about the New Testament authors'.[3]

Thirdly, Bruce J. Malina argues:

If we stick to the earliest traditions in the Gospels, we find it to be quite certain that Jesus proclaimed the kingdom of God and healed people. His healing frequently looked to persons who, in terms of purity rules, were blemished, hence either incapable of social relations with the rest of the holy people of Israel (such as lepers, Mark 1.40–5; Luke 17.11–19; the woman with

[1] Howard Clark Kee, *Medicine, Miracle and Magic in New Testament Times* (Cambridge: Cambridge University Press, 1986), pp. 128–9. See also his *Miracle in the Early Christian World* (New Haven: Yale University Press, 1983), ch. 5.

[2] Gerd Theissen, *The Miracle Stories of the Early Christian Tradition* (Edinburgh and Philadelphia: T. & T. Clark and Fortress Press, 1983; German original 1974), pp. 277–8.

[3] Theissen, *Miracle Stories*, p. 295.

a haemorrhage, Mark 5.25–34) or barred from the Temple and sacrifice because of some sort of permanent impediment or lack of wholeness (such as those possessed, the paralysed, the lame, the blind).[4]

My focus is upon health care in the modern world, so it would be a distraction to trawl through the mass of evidence that all three scholars discuss. It is sufficient for my limited purposes that they conclude so strongly that healing stories reflect the historical ministry of Jesus and occupy such a central role in early Christianity. I will take this as a given, rather than attempt a similar survey myself. My question is simply whether or not the healing stories in the earliest traditions in the Gospels (I will not try to get behind them in a clumsy attempt to reconstruct my own version of the so-called historical Jesus) can provide a distinctive Christian basis for health care ethics in the public forum of a Western, pluralistic society today.

MIRACLES AND HEALING

At once a major difficulty arises. Even in the passages already quoted there are hints about the strangeness for the modern world of these healing stories in the earliest traditions in the Gospels. Both Kee and Theissen, after all, link healings and exorcisms / the casting out of demons and both set the historical Jesus within the apocalyptic tradition. Theissen intensifies this strangeness by referring at times to 'the historical charismatic wonder-worker Jesus'.[5] Malina specifically draws attention to the original context of these stories within Jewish purity rules and temple sacrifice. And both Kee and Theissen warn against appropriating the stories without reflection into modern understandings of healing or health care. A central feature of Kee's book is to distinguish carefully between medicine, miracle and magic. He insists that it is miracle rather than medicine (or magic) that characterises the healing stories in the Gospels:

Indeed, there is in none of these healing stories any trace of medical techniques, and, of course, not a syllable of the language of diagnosis and prescription for disease which we find in the Roman medical tradition of the

---

[4] Bruce J. Malina, *The New Testament World* (Louisville, KY: Westminster John Knox, 3rd edn, 2001), p. 187.
[5] Theissen, *Miracle Stories*, p. 300.

first century . . . the only references to baths in this tradition have to do with ritual cleansings, not with therapy. Neither is there anything that can correctly be labelled magic in these materials. The framework of meaning in which these stories of Jesus' healings are told is not one which assumes that the proper formula or the correct technique will produce the desired results. Rather, the healings and exorcisms are placed in a larger structure which sees what is happening as clues and foretastes of a new situation in which the purpose of God will finally be accomplished in the creation and his people will be vindicated and at peace.[6]

A number of theologians with pastoral concerns have attempted to relate Gospel healing stories, understood primarily as miracles, to modern medicine. Yet they face formidable problems. Two examples, the first from a theological realist tradition and the second from a more purist tradition, can be taken to illustrate this point.

In his 1968 book *Healing Miracles*[7] Hugh Melinsky takes an approach based upon synthesis rather than conflict between healing miracles and modern medicine. He argues at length that David Hume's provocative definition of miracle as 'a violation of the laws of nature' is unsatisfactory in terms both of recent Christian history and of post-Newtonian physics. Rather than being some violation of 'fixed' laws of nature (a concept belonging more to Newton than Einstein) he argues that in recent theology 'miracle is an event which discloses the decisive personal activity of God'.[8] More fully:

First an event is claimed to have happened which does not conform with the normal run of human experience. This is a source of wonder (which is the basic meaning of the word 'miracle'). But, second, in and through this event a claim is made for a particular disclosure of God, his power, his activity, indeed his concern and love. In this respect a miracle is also a sign.[9]

Throughout his study of healing miracles (and in the context of his own extensive experience of hospital chaplaincy) he emphasises that the work of the medical and clerical professions is complementary. He is concerned to challenge scientific reductionism with a reminder that 'man in his wholeness still remains at heart a mystery, and man's

---

[6] Kee, *Medicine, Miracle and Magic*, p. 79.

[7] M. A. H. Melinsky, *Healing Miracles: an Examination from History and Experience of the Place of Miracle in Christian Thought and Medical Practice* (London: Mowbray, 1968).

[8] Melinksy, *Healing Miracles*, p. 178.   [9] Melinksy, *Healing Miracles*, p. 2.

wholeness is now known to be vitally dependent on his relationship with other people, and, Christians would add, with God'.[10] But he is also concerned to warn Christians:

Prayer for the sick is neither a substitute for penicillin nor is it a bludgeoning of God to do what he is otherwise unwilling to do. It is rather an enlarging and deepening of the spiritual-personal realm, a conscious offer of room for the Holy Spirit to move and work in.[11]

Melinsky gives a vivid example from his own experience of the sort of complementary professional relationship that he has in mind. A woman in her forties with severe cancer of the womb and extensive secondary growths was given only weeks to live by her surgeon. Yet in hospital she read the story of the healing of the leper in Mark 1 and began to pray for a healing and knew that others in turn were praying for her. She later wrote to Melinsky that 'during the next few days my worry completely disappeared and I felt a sense of great peace and happiness'.[12] Melinsky was also told by the surgeon that two weeks later he could find no sign of the cancer spreading as had been expected:

I discussed these events with the surgeon at some length, and he confessed to being quite unable to account for her improvement in terms of medical science. He was sure it was not due to the drugs he gave her. He did concede that in his judgement an important factor in her recovery was the spiritual courage with which she faced the knowledge of her condition.[13]

The case seemed to contain both of the criteria in Melinsky's definition of a miracle. In the first place there was something surprising here, both for the surgeon and for the patient, which did not 'conform with the normal run of human experience'. And secondly the patient herself appeared to find in it 'a particular disclosure of God, his power, his activity, indeed his concern and love'.

Yet Melinsky very honestly contains other elements in his account of this case that make the concept of miracle more ambiguous, even troublesome. The woman died a year or so later, albeit facing death with tranquillity. Then, on Melinsky's request, the surgeon wrote this retrospective note:

[10] Melinksy, *Healing Miracles*, p. 109.   [11] Melinsky, *Healing Miracles*, p. 175.
[12] Melinksy, *Healing Miracles*, p. 159.   [13] Melinsky, *Healing Miracles*, p. 160.

In such an apparently hopeless case we thought it worth while trying her on one of the new cytotoxic drugs which have been shown to have a very useful effect against cancer of some types. At the time we had had little experience of the use of this particular drug. Whether it was the result of her knowing exactly how she stood in relation to her life and problems, the result of her own guts in facing up to these problems, or the result of the spiritual assistance which you were able to give her, or indeed the drug itself, remains uncertain; I would like to think a combination of all of them ... I do not think that her apparent improvement was the result of any miracle, because this has been repeated as a result of drug treatment in my later experience; but I still think that the remarkable improvement in her whole mental attitude was a miracle, helped perhaps by myself as well as by you and her faith.[14]

The problem here lies in the first criterion in Melinsky's definition of miracle. In the light of knowledge at the time this was initially an event 'which does not conform with the normal run of human experience'. Yet a subsequent use of cytotoxic drugs on other patients soon rendered it more normal and, with the benefit of hindsight three decades later, actually mundane (as numerous patients have now discovered). Instructively, Aquinas warned that 'when any finite power produces the proper effect to which it is determined, this is not a miracle, though it may be a matter of wonder for some person who does not understand this power ... but what is done by divine power, which, being infinite, is incomprehensible in itself, is truly miraculous'.[15] Melinsky at once admits that the surgeon's note 'shows clearly just how difficult it is to analyse the varied elements in the process of the recovery of a sick person, and how difficult it is, as a result, to be sure of a miraculous element on the physical side'. Then he adds that 'of the miraculous element on the mental or spiritual side in this instance there remains little doubt'.[16]

Herein lies the problem for a book on health care and Christian ethics. The 'wonder' criterion in Melinsky's synthetic understanding of miracles always runs the risk of redundancy. As long as something beneficial in health care 'does not conform with the normal run of

---

[14] Melinksy, *Healing Miracles*, p. 161.
[15] Aquinas, *Summa Contra Gentiles*, trans. Vernon Bourke (London: University of Notre Dame Press and New York: Doubleday, 1975), 3.102–3.
[16] Melinksy, *Healing Miracles*, pp. 161–2.

human experience' it can satisfy the first criterion of what constitutes a miracle. Yet, as medical science and subsequent treatment advance, so what once did not conform with the normal run of human experience may eventually become everyday and mundane instead. Now of course everyday and mundane events can still satisfy the 'sign' criterion, namely that 'in and through this event a claim is made for a particular disclosure of God, his power, his activity, indeed his concern and love'. Many of us do tend to refer to a personally special yet actually ubiquitous event, such as the birth of a baby, as a miracle. But perhaps for most of us this is a self-consciously metaphorical use of the term. It might even be a reminder to the religiously minded that the birth of a baby is one of the great wonders of this God-given world. What we manifestly do not mean is that the birth of a baby 'does not conform with the normal run of human experience'.

The danger for the theologian here is that any distinctive insight that she/he has to offer is squeezed into a tighter and tighter corner. As medical science becomes ever better at providing adequate explanations for particular diseases, as well as finding effective cures for them, so even a synthetic understanding of healing miracles tends to become superfluous. Or, to put this another way, the original judgement of the surgeon in Melinsky's case study that a miracle may have taken place, effecting a physical cure for the woman from her cancer, gave way to a more metaphorical invocation of a 'miraculous' change of attitude, and then perhaps to a blunter conviction that it was chemotherapy alone that accounted for her temporary physical remission.

Melinsky himself is sensitive to this dilemma and treads very cautiously. His central concern (like my own) is to work as a priest and theologian alongside health care professionals – taking their role seriously while not surrendering the distinctiveness of his own. Yet the concept of 'miracles' threatens to disrupt this relationship. Healing miracles viewed as 'a violation of the laws of nature' threaten serious conflict. However healing miracles viewed in synthetic terms become ever more redundant as medical knowledge advances. In the context of mainstream Western health care, an approach based upon healing miracles seems to offer the prospect of either conflict or slow, ineluctable retreat.

Writing from a more purist theological stance, Colin Brown also detects dangers in this area. Like Melinsky, he rejects Hume's understanding of miracles as 'a violation of the laws of nature', arguing instead that 'perhaps the time has come for us to listen more attentively to the witness of Augustine, Calvin, and Luther ... we might find ourselves asking whether we need to look beyond the apparent violation of nature to the harmony of a higher order'.[17] In his writings Brown emphasises that belief in miracles has never been straightforward for Christians, pointing out, for example, that Luther argued that 'the day of miracles is past' and that in any event miracles are 'the least significant works, since they are only physical and are performed for only a few people'.[18] After making a wide-ranging historical survey Brown himself concludes that 'testimony to the miraculous was no less difficult to believe for the educated person in the second century than for his or her twentieth-century counterpart'.[19]

Brown writes from an explicitly Christian evangelical commitment. Nevertheless, he is particularly critical of fellow evangelicals who argue for what they term 'covenanted healing':

Many bereaved people are prone to depression and guilt because of the nagging feeling that they did not love enough or care enough for the one whom they have now lost. If the bereaved are taught that God has covenanted to heal those who are prayed for in faith, this depression and guilt can be intensified. It can make them feel that they are personally responsible for the death of their loved one because they did not pray enough or believe enough. Instead of finding comfort and hope in the assurances of God's gift of eternal life to those who turn to him, such people can be subjected to the Satanic temptation to self-recrimination and despair.[20]

Significantly, it seems to be pastoral experience that makes Brown, like Melinsky, cautious here. If too much is claimed for healing miracles in the context of health care today, then there is a real risk not just of disappointment but of deep shame as well. The person of faith *knows* that she/he or a loved one will be cured if only she/he has

[17] Colin Brown, *That You May Believe: Miracles and Faith Then and Now* (Grand Rapids, MI: William B. Eerdmans, 1985), p. 16.

[18] *Luther's Works* ed., Jaroslav Pelikan (St Louis, MO: Concordia, 1961), 24:79.

[19] Colin Brown, *Miracles and the Critical Mind* (Grand Rapids, MI: William B. Eerdmans, 1984), p. 18.

[20] Brown, *That You May Believe*, p. 204.

sufficient faith. So when no cure happens, the person is likely to see this not just as an absence of cure but, more disturbingly, as an indictment of her/his faith. Brown might also have added at this point that such expectations are likely to affect the healer as well. Those healers who make strong claims for covenanted healing are themselves under considerable pressure to deliver demonstrable 'cures'. It is hardly surprising, then, that there have been so many charges of delusion or chicanery in this area.

Like Melinsky again, Brown is anxious not to disrupt modern, professional health care with exaggerated claims about 'covenanted healing':

One special danger that may come if we assume that God has covenanted to heal everyone if only he or she has enough faith is the danger that we make faith a substitute for proper care and medical attention. Hardly a month passes that the news media do not give a report of some tragic case in which someone has made the mistake of assuming faith was an adequate alternative to proper medical care ... What must be questioned is the folly of thinking that faith requires us to abandon the means God has provided for the well-being of humankind.[21]

The radical logic of the 'covenanted healing' position is that all healing should be left to faith. Once it is fervently believed that 'God has covenanted to heal everyone if only he or she has enough faith', then any resort to modern, professional health care would seem to be superfluous. For those who truly believe in 'covenanted healing', mundane forms of health care would, at best, appear to be redundant. Such mundane forms are no longer needed when compared with the miraculous healing power that God alone can provide.

At worst, any resort to mundane health care could be seen as an indication that the person, although theoretically committed to 'covenanted healing', does not in reality have enough faith. After all, the conditional clause in Brown's understanding of 'covenanted healing' is 'if only he or she has enough faith'. There is a clear warning here which has bedevilled many such Christians. Manifestly not all those who are prayed for (by Christians of any variety) do recover from their illness. A less evangelical Christian is likely to recognise

---

[21] Brown, *That You May Believe*, p. 205.

this, adding 'but thy will be done' to any intercessionary prayer. In contrast, those committed to 'covenanted healing' believe that if only they have enough faith then the ill will be cured. So when inevitably some, or even many, of the ill are not cured or even die, the obvious explanation for this is that someone (whether those praying or even the ill person herself) did not have enough faith. And one clear indication that that is so is that the person herself, or others on her behalf, resorted to mundane health care. The latter ought (logically at least) to be unnecessary for believers in 'covenanted healing' and might actually be sinful since it indicates that something other than pure faith is needed for a cure to be effected.

It is not necessary to claim that all of those committed to 'covenanted healing' in reality view mundane health care as either redundant or sinful. In practice most of us live with contradictions in our everyday life, not least in areas of vulnerability such as illness and mortality. Few follow the radical (and logical) path of, say, Christian Scientists. Rather it is the internal logic of 'covenanted healing' which suggests this conclusion and which may generate special (theo)logical problems for those Christians committed to such healing.

So an impasse seems to be reached. The abundant stories of healing in the Synoptic Gospels, which at first appear to offer such an attractive basis for a distinctively Christian ethical commentary on healing and health in the modern world, are derailed by the miraculous. The scepticism about seeking to combine the strange world of the New Testament with realities in the modern world does seem to be justified. Theological purists who do so in the context of modern, secular health care are set on a course of serious collision, whereas theological realists who do so find themselves defending a smaller and smaller territory. Is this the only choice?

HEALING AND CURING

John Pilch's work offers a rather different approach. In a series of articles[22] and in his fascinating book *Healing in the New*

---

[22] E.g. John Pilch, 'Understanding Healing in the Social World of Early Christianity', *Biblical Theology Bulletin*, 22:1 (1992), pp. 26–33 (see his bibliography for other articles by him going back to 1981).

*Testament: Insights from Medical and Mediterranean Anthropology*²³ he
sets the healing stories into a fresh context. Appropriating insights
from medical anthropology, he seeks to show how health and sickness,
and then suitable therapies, are variously understood in different
cultures. In the process he is able to demonstrate important points of
comparison as well as contrast between modern medicine and healing
in New Testament times.

He makes a fundamental distinction between 'healing' and 'cure':

In Western, scientifically-oriented cultures, therapies are aetiological, that
is, they focus on the causes of diseases: germs or viruses . . . Clearly such a
situation requires the existence of a microscope and a host of other relatively
recent inventions, technologies, and the like. The name given to this specific
kind of therapy is *cure*, that is, the taking of effective control of a disordered
biological and/or psychological process, usually identified as a *disease* . . . In
cultures that are not scientifically oriented, therapies are symptomatic, that
is, aimed at alleviating or managing the symptoms. This process invariably
entails creating new meaning for the sufferer . . . The name given to this
kind of therapy is *healing*, namely 'a process by which (a) disease and certain
other worrisome circumstances are made into illness (a cultural construction
and therefore meaningful), and (b) the sufferer gains a degree of satisfaction through the reduction, or even the elimination of the psychological,
sensory, and experiential oppressiveness engendered by his medical
circumstances'.²⁴

Expressed like this the contrast between 'cure' and 'healing' – the
first representing the modern world and the second the New
Testament world – functions almost as an ideal type in Pilch's
writings. He is well aware, for example, that not everything that
happens in Western medicine today is aetiological and that medical
practice is not always about 'cure' rather than 'healing'. Rather it is
that aetiology and cure are the ultimate aims of Western medicine
and practice. In contrast, the fundamental aims and assumptions of
healing in the New Testament (and in the ancient world generally)
are radically different. Viewed in summary terms, Western medicine
is primarily concerned with: doing or achieving; individualism;

²³ John Pilch, *Healing in the New Testament: Insights from Medical and Mediterranean
   Anthropology* (Minneapolis: Fortress Press, 2000).
²⁴ Pilch, *Healing in the NT*, pp. 13–14 (Pilch is quoting from Arthur Kleinman, *Patients and
   Healers in the Context of Culture*, Berkeley: University of California Press, 1980, p. 265).

future-orientation; mastery over nature; and views human nature as good or neutral and thus correctable. In similar summary terms, New Testament healing is primarily concerned with: being and/or becoming; collateral or linear relationships; present and past time orientation; and views nature as uncontrollable and human nature as both good and bad.

On the basis of this distinction he is amazed at fellow Christians today who go to their doctors requiring aetiological medicine, based upon properly scientific investigations, and yet who go to church and treat healing stories in the Gospels at face value as 'cures' but without being able to make any similar investigations. In contrast, he insists that:

The sickness problems presented to Jesus in the New Testament are concerned with a state of being (blind; deaf; mute; leprosy [an 'unclean' skin condition rather than Hansen's disease]; death; uncontrolled haemorrhaging, rather than an inability to function. What a Western reader might interpret as a loss of function, namely lameness, an ancient reader would see as a disvalued state of being. This is expressed in the Levitical code where, among those descendants of Aaron who may not offer the bread, it lists: 'a man blind or lame, or one who has a mutilated face or a limb too long, or a man who has an injured foot or an injured hand' (Lev. 21:18–19). Thus the real problem for the paralytics in the Synoptics (Mark 2:1–11 and parallels) and in John 5 is not their obvious inability to do something, but their disvalued state.[25]

Here, of course, there is a point of contact between the ancient and modern worlds. Manifestly not all surgery today is aimed at restoring function. Cosmetic surgery, for example, is much more to do with 'being' than 'doing' and is frequently about 'disvalued states'.

Pilch's aim is not to make the healing stories in the Gospels redundant in the modern world, but rather to understand them better and to help 'an interpreter to be a respectful reader of biblical material'.[26] In a poignant conclusion to his book he tells of how his wife died recently from ovarian cancer. After initial surgery she was told by her surgeon that she was definitely in remission. She asked him: 'Do you mean that I am cured?' But he responded quite

---

[25] Pilch, *Healing in the NT*, p. 13.   [26] Pilch, *Healing in the NT*, p. 116.

properly: 'We can't use that word until you are in remission for five years.' In the event she only lived for three. Pilch comments:

As modern Western medicine admits, cure is a relatively rare occurrence in human experience. For most of the twentieth century, human sickness has peaked and subsided before modern medicine discovered a cure. Often the human body accommodates and learns how to defeat the sickness. In some cases this takes longer than in others. Healing, on the other hand, occurs always, infallibly, 100 per cent of the time. Healing is the restoration of meaning to life. All people, no matter how serious their condition, eventually come to some resolution. My wife was healed even before she went into remission and continued in her healed state until she died. She and I discovered new meaning in life, meaning specific to this shared experience of battling the disease, and ultimately – in our case – recognizing that the disease had won.[27]

This account is very close to the one offered by Melinsky, yet there are two crucial differences. Melinsky continues to talk about the 'miraculous' in his account and appears to move from an initial belief that some miraculous physical cure had been effected to a more spiritual interpretation instead. Pilch makes no mention of the miraculous here and distinguishes between 'cure' and 'healing'. Nevertheless the end result of the two accounts is remarkably similar. Both of these experienced pastors are convinced that the two women involved underwent a genuine restoration of meaning and spirit before they died from the physical effects of ovarian cancer. Even for Pilch, 'healing' in this sense seems finally to take precedent over physical cure – despite the fact that the sights of Western medicine are so firmly set at such cure.

The fresh perspective that Pilch offers is helpful, but only up to a point, for a study of *Health Care and Christian Ethics*. His focus upon 'healing' rather than miracle in the Gospel stories is particularly helpful. Too many other biblical commentators have done little more than discuss rival understandings of 'miracle' in relation to these stories. Doubtless there is a proper place for this within broader philosophical and theological considerations. Yet, as already argued, within the narrow concerns of professional health care today miracles soon become an obstacle or a distraction. Again, Pilch's judicious use

[27] Pilch, *Healing in the NT*, p. 141.

of social science as a means of understanding the context of these stories, albeit without eliminating their theological significance, is also helpful. The discussions within medical anthropology about cultural differences and similarities do help to avoid the conflations between healing within the New Testament and modern medicine against which both Theissen and Kee warn. The specific distinction between 'healing' and 'cure' is also helpful. He is certainly not suggesting that modern medicine should abandon its quest for 'cure', based upon aetiological diagnosis and functional therapy, and return instead to New Testament 'healing'. But he is saying that the latter can add an important dimension even to our understanding of health in the modern world. 'Healing' – properly understood as a complement, not an alternative, to modern medicine – is still available to people in the twenty-first century even in the absence of 'cure'.

HEALING VIRTUES

Yet the concern of the present study is wider than this. The concern here is to identify, if possible, specifically Christian resources that might make a distinctive contribution to health care ethics today in the public forum of a Western, pluralistic society. This is not exactly Pilch's concern, so it would be unfair to criticise him for not addressing it. How might such resources be identified from the healing stories in the Synoptic Gospels?

One obvious way would be to analyse these stories for the explicit or implicit virtues that they might contain. Here too the skills of the social scientist might be helpful. Identifying implicit assumptions, beliefs and practices – sometimes at odds with those that are explicitly stated – is germane to social science. Both quantitative and qualitative methods can be used to achieve this in the modern world, as I attempted to demonstrate at length in *Churchgoing and Christian Ethics.*[28] In the ancient world it is likely to be qualitative methods alone that are appropriate. However, by using such methods

---

[28] Robin Gill, *Churchgoing and Christian Ethics* (Cambridge: Cambridge University Press, 1999).

effectively it might be possible to analyse the healing stories in the Synoptic Gospels to uncover the virtues implicit within them.

Qualitative methods in social science typically look for regularities and correlations. So qualitative research using extended interviews with subjects is often based upon a loosely structured framework (allowing, as far as possible, subjects to express their thoughts on a particular topic using their own words). The interviews are recorded and then transcribed. In turn, the transcriptions can be analysed (often using an appropriate software program) in order to see which explicit words or phrases – or implicit notions – occur or are combined most regularly within the transcriptions. Qualitative research of this sort lacks the 'objectivity' of randomised, stratified quantitative sampling. Yet it gains a depth and specificity that would otherwise not be possible. Individual subjects can be given a real opportunity to express themselves in their own terms and not simply in those of the interviewers.

Empirical research using such qualitative methods often focuses upon details within a recorded interview or written story that might otherwise appear trivial. Social anthropologists and qualitative sociologists are trained to look beyond public explanations, in the belief both that human beings have complex forms of behaviour of which they are only partially aware and that interpersonal communication usually consists of more than verbal expressions. For example, those social scientists who are trained to observe non-verbal body language learn to identify patterns of social communication among human subjects who are themselves largely unconscious of these patterns. Seemingly trivial gestures, body movements, eye contact and non-verbal noises are used by these social scientists as evidence of complex forms of social communication. Indeed, among those people with Asperger's Syndrome it is often these seemingly trivial gestures, movements and noises that are either absent in their social interactions or are present but in forms that are unfamiliar to most other people. So although some of those with this syndrome may be highly skilled in verbal logic, other people may be confused by the asymmetry between their verbal and non-verbal skills of communication. They literally 'send out mixed messages'.

If the healing stories within the texts of the earliest Gospel traditions are inspected in this way, what patterns of reported behaviour – or, more specifically, what values or virtues – recur? Caution is needed at this point. Vernon Robbins reminds the incautious that 'there is not simply a text; texts were produced by authors and they are meaningless without readers. There are not simply readers; readers are meaningless without texts to read and authors who write texts. All three presuppose historical, social, cultural and ideological relations among people and the texts they write and read.'[29] In the light of the considerable advances of biblical interpretation over the last two decades, it would be naïve to claim that any focus upon particular biblical texts – let alone my own – is free from an element of 'reader response'. My own focus here is quite explicit – namely a concern for healing within the context of Western medicine. Any focus of this sort inevitably involves some 'historical, social, cultural and ideological relation' between myself and the Synoptic texts.

Nonetheless, some approximate way of counting might help to identify the most prevalent patterns that are actually present within these texts whether or not it is me that is involved in the study of them. It would be a mistake to attempt to turn this into a formal, quantitative exercise. The very nature of the Synoptic Gospels precludes this, since they contain so much duplicate material as well as variant textual readings. In any case it is sometimes a matter of personal judgement whether or not a particular virtue is thought to be implicit within a particular story. At most any system of counting is a means of identifying rough prevalence. With this in mind, the system used here will be to give a full weighting to a primary occurrence in one of the Synoptic sources and just half a weighting for a parallel occurrence (judging the latter to be not without significance yet not as significant as the former).

Passionate emotion is a very strong feature of the Synoptic healing stories. This takes several forms: sometimes it is Jesus being portrayed as angry; sometimes it is the healing being set in a situation of sharp confrontation; and sometimes it is the crowd which is portrayed as being afraid or amazed. In all of these forms taken together (and they do often occur together) passionate emotion has a very high rating of some eighteen. Crowd amazement/fear occurs usually at the end of

[29] Vernon Robbins, *The Tapestry of Early Christian Discourse: Rhetoric, Society and Ideology* (London: Routledge, 1996), p. 39.

a number of stories in Mark: the man in the synagogue (1.27), the paralytic (2.12), the Gadarene demoniac (5.15), Jairus' daughter (5.42) and the deaf-mute (7.37). Matthew and/or Luke have parallels with all of these stories and in addition share a further story of the blind/ dumb demoniac (Matt. 12.23 / Luke 11.14). Matthew also has a crowd 'wondering' (15.31) and Luke has a crowd afraid (after the raising of the widow of Nain's son in 7.16). Sharp controversy also features in several healing stories: sometimes because the healing is on a Sabbath – the man with the withered hand (Mark 3.1–6 / Matt. 12.9–14 / Luke 6.6–11) and in Luke's stories of the woman with an eighteen-year infirmity (13.10–21) and the man with dropsy (14.1–6); on another occasion the sharp controversy involves supposed healing by Beelzebub (Matt. 12.22–32 / Luke 11.14–20); and on another it is about the power to forgive sins (Mark 2.3–12 / Matt. 9.2–8 / Luke 5.18–26). Jesus himself variously shows anger or compassion, according to differing texts, towards the leper in Mark (1.43), anger towards the Pharisees in the story of the man with the withered hand (3.5), and in Matthew the two blind men are told 'sternly' by Jesus to tell no one (9.30).

Faith (with a weighting of some fifteen) is another very strong feature in the Synoptic healing stories. The phrase 'your faith has made you well', said by Jesus directly to the one who has just been healed, is addressed in all three Gospels to the woman with a haemorrhage (Mark 5.34 / Matt. 9.22 / Luke 8.48), in Mark and Luke to blind Bartimaeus (Mark 10.52 / Luke 18.42) and in Luke alone to one of the ten lepers (17.19). In a Matthew story (9.28) Jesus asks the two blind men 'Do you believe that I am able to do this' before healing them, whereas in Mark's story of the epileptic boy (9.24) it is the father who declares 'I believe, help my unbelief' before his son is healed. In a number of other healing stories Jesus recognises the faith of those close to the one who was to be healed: the paralytic man in all three Gospels (Mark 2.5 / Matt. 9.2 / Luke 5.20), the centurion's servant in Matthew and Luke (Matt. 8.10 / Luke 7.9), and in Matthew's version of the Marcan story of the Canaanite woman (15.28). A lack of faith on the part of the would-be healer is given as the reason in all three Gospels for the inability of the disciples to heal the epileptic boy (Mark 9.19 / Matt. 17.17 / Luke 9.41) and a lack of faith by others is associated in Mark and Matthew with Jesus' inability to heal many in his home country (Mark 6.5–6 / Matt. 13.58).

Mercy or compassion features in several forms within the Synoptic healing stories (with a weighting of at least fourteen). The most common of these is for a story to begin with a plea to Jesus for mercy from the ill or their relatives. This form can be found explicitly in Mark's story of blind Bartimaeus (Mark 10.47 / Luke 18.37) and in both of Matthew's parallel stories of two blind men (9.27 and 20.30); in Luke's story of the ten lepers (17.13); in Matthew's versions of the Canaanite/Syro-Phoenician woman (15.22) and the epileptic boy (17.15). An initial plea for mercy may also be present implicitly in those stories which involve people begging Jesus and/or prostrating themselves before him asking for a healing: in all three Gospels the leper (Mark 1.40 / Matt. 8.2 / Luke 5.11) and Jairus (Mark 5.22–3 / Matt. 9.18 / Luke 8.41), and in Mark the Syro-Phoenician woman (7.26) and the blind man at Bethsaida (8.22). In Mark's original story of the epileptic, the boy's father asks Jesus not for 'mercy' but for 'pity' or 'compassion' (9.22) – using the verb *splankgnizesthai* rather than *eleos* (mercy). In a number of stories it is compassion that is explicitly attributed to Jesus himself: in Luke's story of the widow at Nain (7.13); in two of Matthew's accounts of crowds associated with healing (9.36 and 14.14); and in some texts of Mark's story of the leper (1.41). In Matthew's story of the two blind men at Jericho (20.29–34) 'mercy' and 'compassion' uniquely are both used: the blind men cry to Jesus 'Have mercy on us' and again 'Lord, have mercy on us' and Jesus responds in 'compassion' touching their eyes. In a context of care, rather than healing as such, 'compassion' is attributed to Jesus as a reason for the feeding of the four thousand in both Mark and Matthew (Mark 8.2 / Matt. 15.32) and the feeding of the five thousand in Mark (6.34). Compassion also features at pivotal points in Luke's parables of the good Samaritan (10.33) and prodigal son (15.20) and in Matthew's parable of the unmerciful servant (18.27).

Another prevalent feature of the healing stories (with an overall weighting of at least twelve) involves touching. Jesus touching the person to be healed is a very strong feature indeed. In Mark alone Jesus touches Peter's mother-in-law (1.31), the leper (1.41), Jairus' daughter (5.41), some sick people (6.5), the deaf-mute (7.33), the blind man (8.23) and the epileptic boy (9.27). Two of these stories have parallels in Matthew and Luke and a further one in Matthew but not Luke. In addition, Luke has two separate stories involving Jesus touching – the bier of the widow's son (7.14) and the woman with an eighteen-year infirmity (13.13) – and Matthew tells of Jesus touching two blind men (9.29). In addition to all of these reports of touching there are two other stories – the woman with the haemorrhage (Mark 5.27 / Matt. 9.20 / Luke 8.44) and the crowd at Gennesaret (Mark 6.56 / Matt. 14.36) – in which the people to be healed touch Jesus' garments.

A related feature, namely uncleanness, is explicitly linked to two of these stories – the leper, found in all three Gospels, and the epileptic boy, in Mark alone – and may be implicitly present in several more of the stories. The overall prevalence weighting for uncleanness/cleansing is almost as high as for touching. So in Mark it also features in the man in the synagogue (1.23 and 27), the crowd (3.11), the Gadarene demoniac (5.2 and 13) and the Syro-Phoenician woman's daughter (7.25). Luke has parallels with the first three of these and an additional story featuring cleansing – the ten lepers (17.14). Matthew also has Jesus' command to the twelve disciples to 'cleanse lepers' (10.8).

A feature of healing stories that has attracted much scholarly attention during the last century is reticence or restraint (with a weighting of around ten). Jesus gives a command at the end of several stories that no one should be told: in Mark and Luke he commands cast-out demons not to speak (Mark 1.34 / Luke 4.41); in all three Gospels (Mark 1.44 / Matt. 8.4 / Luke 5.14) he tells the leper to tell no one (with Mark including the adverb 'sternly'); in Mark he orders unclean spirits not to make him known and in the parallel Matthew story he gives the same order to those that have been healed (Mark 3.12 / Matt. 12.16); in Mark and Luke he tells Jairus and his family to tell no one after his daughter has been healed (Mark 5.43 / Luke 8.56); in Mark Jesus charges people more than once to tell no one after the healing of the deaf-mute (7.36) and tells the blind man 'Do not even enter the village' after his healing (8.26); and in Matthew Jesus 'sternly' charges the two blind men 'See that no one knows it' (9.30). This feature of reticence or restraint is not wholly consistent. For instance, Jesus tells unclean spirits in Mark and Luke to be silent (Mark 1.25 / Luke 4.35), but in the same Gospels the Gadarene demoniac once healed is told to go home and tell what 'the Lord' (in Mark) or 'God' (in Luke) 'has done for you' (Mark 5.19 / Luke 8.39). In addition, in both Matthew and Luke Jesus uses his healings as evidence for John the Baptist (Matt. 11.4–5 / Luke 7.22) and in Luke for Herod (13.32).

Although these are all frequent within the Synoptic healing stories, there are other features that occur but less often. Ironically, such minority features have sometimes been given particular attention within biblical commentaries. For example, only in Matthew and Luke is a direct link made between healing and the Kingdom of God (Matt. 12.28 / Luke 11.20) and even within these two Gospels this link is most unusual. Again, an explicit identification of healing as a 'sign' is a feature of John (4.54) rather than the Synoptic Gospels. Yet considerable attention has been given to both of these features in discussions of healing stories within the Synoptic Gospels. Another feature that has received considerable attention is the use of Aramaic commands at the very moment of healing. For example, it encouraged early form critics to identify this as a magical technique similar to other ancient miracle stories. It is indeed a feature of two of Mark's stories (5.41 and 7.34), but it does not occur in parallels or elsewhere in the Synoptic healing stories and may be explained simply as being appropriate to their original context (as in 3.17, 7.11, 14.36, 15.22 and 15.34).[30] In Mark there are a number of other links that are occasionally made: synagogues feature in five of the healing stories (1.23, 1.39, 3.1, 5.36 and 6.2), 'authority' is explicit in three stories (1.27, 2.10 and 3.15), sin and forgiveness in one (2.5–10), power in another (5.30) and 'prayer' in yet another (9.29). It certainly must not be assumed that these less frequent features are unimportant. However, a qualitative approach to evidence does carry an *a priori* assumption that if features regularly and spontaneously recur within interviews or written stories, then they may well be an indication of values or commitments that might otherwise be overlooked. On this basis particular attention needs to be given to those six features – passionate emotion,

---

[30] See further Vincent Taylor, *The Gospel According to St Mark* (London: Macmillan, 1959), p. 296, and Morna D. Hooker, *The Gospel According to St Mark* (London: A. & C. Black, 1991), p. 150.

faith, mercy/compassion, touching, uncleanness and reticence/restraint – that occur most often in the Synoptic healing stories.

So far these six features have been discussed in the order of their rough prevalence. Given the crude way that their different weightings have been measured, this is hardly satisfactory. All that has been established up to this point is that it is these features – rather than a link with the Kingdom of God, signs, Aramaic commands, synagogues, authority, sin/forgiveness, power or prayer – which are the most characteristic features of the Synoptic healing stories. It might, though, be more logical to order these most characteristic features in terms of their sequence actually within healing stories. On this basis, mercy/compassion typically occurs at the beginning of stories, faith soon after the healing and reticence/restraint at the end. The remaining features – passionate emotion, touching and uncleanness – tend to cluster in association in the middle of healing stories. An overall four-fold pattern begins to emerge: an initial plea for mercy/compassion, followed by passionate emotion/unclean touching – *then the healing itself* – followed by a recognition of faith, and concluding with a command for restraint.

In sociological terms this is an 'ideal' typology (or, in Wittgenstein's philosophical terms, 'family resemblance'): it depicts the characteristic pattern of a Synoptic healing but not the actual pattern of any particular story. Only in the combined stories of the healing of Jairus' daughter and the woman with a haemorrhage can all four elements be found: the prostrate opening plea of Jairus / the weeping and wailing in Jairus' house, the touching of the daughter by Jesus and the unclean touching of Jesus by the woman / the faith of the woman / and the command to Jairus and his family to tell no one. All of the Synoptic stories contain at least one (and usually more) of the four, but none contains them all.

COMPASSION

A plea for mercy/compassion typically initiates a healing story. Melinsky states bluntly and inaccurately:

To attempt to understand the healing miracles in terms of nineteenth-century philanthropy is to try measuring a patient's temperature with a slide-rule. In fact, compassion for a sick person is never in the gospels a primary motive for Jesus' healing.[31]

He forgets, of course, Matthew's accounts of Jesus' response to crowds seeking healing (9.36 and 14.14), his story of the two blind men (20.34) and Luke's story of the widow at Nain (7.13) (Melinsky, in line with Vincent Taylor, discounts the variant reading in Mark 1.41). However, even biblical commentators have been apt to play down the role of compassion in the Synoptic healing stories. So, all that A. H. M'Neile comments on Matt. 20.34 is: 'An expression of emotion in Matt., absent from Mark, is unusual',[32] and all that C. F. Evans comments on Luke 7.13 is: 'Only here and Matt. 20.34 as the motive for performing a miracle.'[33]

Given the combined evidence within the earliest Gospel traditions just rehearsed – including explicit and implicit pleas for mercy alongside direct depictions of Jesus' compassion – this does seem to be too narrow an interpretation. It is interesting that in the second edition of his influential book *Conflict, Holiness and Politics in the Teaching of Jesus*, one of the major changes that Marcus Borg makes is to change 'mercy' and 'merciful' to 'compassion' and 'compassionate':

The justification for the change is very simple. Namely the most common connotations of 'mercy' and 'merciful' in modern English do not express the meanings of the relevant gospel and biblical texts. In English 'mercy' and 'merciful' commonly have two closely related dimensions of meaning. First, showing mercy typically presumes a situation of wrongdoing. One is merciful to somebody who has done wrong ... Second, the language of mercy commonly presumes a power relationship of superior to inferior ... But in most synoptic contexts, these meanings are not only not called for, but are often inappropriate. The word 'compassion' avoids these connotations. As its Latin roots suggest, compassion means 'to feel with'. To be compassionate means to feel the feelings of another, and then to act accordingly.[34]

[31] Melinsky, *Healing Miracles*, p. 18.

[32] A. H. M'Neile, *The Gospel According to St Matthew* (London and New York: Macmillan and St Martin's Press, 1965), p. 292.

[33] C. F. Evans, *Saint Luke* (London and Philadelphia: SCM Press and Trinity Press, 1990), p. 348.

[34] Marcus J. Borg, *Conflict, Holiness and Politics in the Teaching of Jesus* (Harrisburg, PA: Trinity Press International, 2nd edn, 1998), p. 16.

Even in the later traditions of healing stories to be found in John and Acts compassion does not seem to be absent: in John, Jesus responds to the official who begs him to come down and heal his son (4.47) and is reported at the outset of the Lazarus story to 'love' Martha, Mary and Lazarus (11.5), and, in Acts, the first healing story is depicted by Peter as 'a good deed' (4.9). Compassion does seem to be more significant in the early Christian narratives than some allow.

CARE

After compassion in the Synoptic healing stories comes a cluster of actions and attitudes which collectively, and in the context of health today, might most appropriately be termed 'care'. This term embraces actions as well as attitudes in that, properly understood, it involves both 'caring for' and 'caring about' those in need.

This combination of caring for and caring about is apparent in a number of the healing stories, but it is particularly a feature of Mark's versions of the healing of the leper (1.40–5) and the epileptic boy (9.14–29). Placed so early in Mark's Gospel, the story of the leper contains a powerful combination of Jesus deliberately touching someone who is deemed to be ritually unclean with deep emotions attributed to Jesus in the course of this healing. As Morna Hooker maintains:

The significance of the story lies in Jesus' amazing power to heal even this condition. To us, leprosy seems the most loathsome of diseases; to the Jew, it was also the most strident example of uncleanness. Whether or not the so-called leper was suffering from what we should recognize as a contagious disease, he was certainly *regarded* as contagious: he was not allowed to come into contact with other human beings or with their property and was thus totally cut off from society. In touching this man, Jesus did not simply run the risk of catching leprosy, but he also made himself unclean according to the regulations of the Mosaic Law. Yet the outcome of the story is not that Jesus is made unclean, but that the leper is made clean![35]

Unlike the parallel stories in Matthew and Luke, the story in Mark contains three separate words ('anger' or 'compassion' in verse 41 and 'stern' and 'sent away' in verse 45) 'which suggest agitation or strong

[35] Hooker, *The Gospel According to St Mark*, pp. 78–9.

emotion in Jesus' part'. Only John's powerful account of Jesus' emotions at the centre of the Lazarus story (11.33–8) can rival this. As a result Hooker argues that 'it is probable that Mark himself understood Jesus' anger and emotion as caused by the forces of evil and disease with which he is here in conflict'.[36]

A combination of anger and touching someone who is unclean is also a strong feature of the story of the epileptic boy. In Mark Jesus 'rebuked the unclean spirit' (9.25) and then took the boy 'by the hand and lifted him up' (9.27). However, the story also starts with controversy involving the scribes, as well as the crowd, for once, 'amazed' at the outset (9.15). And Jesus, in turn, is angry in this unusually long story for Mark, apparently with the disciples, denouncing them in all three Gospels as 'O faithless generation' (9.19).

Caring about those in need properly involves attention to their social and physical context as well as to their immediate cause of concern. In chapter 5 it will be seen that an approach to health care based upon what is now termed systems pastoral care involves attention to the patient as a person rather than just to her/his particular disease. That is exactly what is denoted by the passionate emotions depicted in the Synoptic healing stories. Sometimes these emotions are directed at the disease itself or at the 'unclean spirits'. Yet at other times they involve the faithlessness of the disciples or the religious authorities of the time. Even the crowd emotions, which more typically come at the end of a healing story (as in Luke 9.43), can be a source of concern to Jesus. The early narrative in Mark is punctuated with crowd-induced difficulties for Jesus: 'Jesus could no longer openly enter a town' (1.45); 'Jesus withdrew with his disciples to the sea, and a great multitude from Galilee followed' (3.7); and he withdrew in a boat 'lest they should crush him; for he had healed many, so that all who had diseases pressed upon him to touch him' (3.9–10).

FAITH

The third feature in the healing stories – faith – is multi-layered as well, both within the Synoptic Gospels and (implicitly) within modern health care. At first sight the frequent mention of faith

[36] Hooker, *The Gospel According to St Mark*, p. 81.

within the Synoptic stories might seem to be the least relevant of the four features to a modern pluralistic society. However, chapter 6 will argue that, properly understood again, it remains a very important, albeit neglected, feature of health care ethics and that the latter is impoverished if the various layers of faith within a healing relationship are ignored.

At the most basic level the 'faith' required of those to be healed (or their families/friends) in the Synoptic stories appears to be a faithful trust in Jesus as healer. In the later traditions of healing stories in John and Acts *pistis* is clearly more than this: in a context of healing, people become 'believers' (e.g. John 4.53 and Acts 5.14) and *pistis* is explicitly in Jesus or in his name (e.g. John 11.25 and Acts 3.16). Yet in the Synoptic stories faith appears more ambiguous and commentators tend to have different ways of interpreting it (doubtless reflecting their own particular theological positions or 'reader responses'). For example, among those commentators concerned primarily with *pistis* in the healing stories in Mark: for Vincent Taylor it primarily 'denotes a confident trust in Jesus and in his power to help';[37] for J. M. Robinson 'Mark has no single person or act as the object of faith, and no specific credal statement as the content of faith. Rather it is faith in the action recorded in Marcan history';[38] Christopher D. Marshall, in contrast, considers that Robinson 'is much too vague, for the object of faith is, in a sense, quite specific: the presence of God's eschatological power in the person of Jesus'[39] (but note here Marshall's phrase 'in a sense', especially since he has earlier admitted to 'some ambiguity concerning the intended object of faith'[40]). Among commentators more widely there are also differences: for A. H. M'Neile *pistis* is 'not belief in Him as divine, but confidence that He could perform a miracle';[41] for Davies and Allison it is 'belief in Jesus and his power as miracle worker';[42] and for C. F. Evans it is simply 'confidence in Jesus as the source of power'.[43] Despite these

[37] Taylor, *The Gospel According to St Mark*, p. 194.

[38] J. M. Robinson, *The Problem of History in Mark* (London: SCM Press, 1957), p. 13.

[39] Christopher D. Marshall, *Faith as a Theme in Mark's Narrative* (Cambridge: Cambridge University Press, 1989), p. 232.

[40] Marshall, *Faith*, p. 230.   [41] M'Neile, *The Gospel According to St Matthew*, p. 105.

[42] W. D. Davies and Dale C. Allison Jr, *A Critical Commentary on The Gospel According to Saint Matthew*, vol. II (Edinburgh: T. & T. Clark, 1991), p. 25.

[43] Evans, *Saint Luke*, p. 391.

differences there does seem to be widespread agreement that *pistis* here has less to do with confessional belief, let alone intellectual assent (as in Mark 13.21), than with trust/confidence.

It is certainly a feature of several of the Synoptic healing stories that faith is demonstrated by action rather than declared verbally, and it is not always even the one to be healed who actually does this demonstrating. So in the story of the paralytic man in Mark and Luke it seems to have been the determined action of friends which was responsible for Jesus seeing their faith (Mark 2.5 / Luke 5.20). Commentators have again differed among themselves about whether or not the paralytic man was included in the faith that Jesus saw. There is obviously no way of telling what the Gospel writers themselves intended here (let alone what happened in reality). In any case in those stories involving someone presumed to be dead her/his faith was clearly not involved. Another instance of determined but silent action, in all three Gospels here, followed by Jesus' commendation of faith, is the woman with a haemorrhage (or, perhaps more accurately, with ritually unclean vaginal bleeding). In Mark and Matthew, significantly, the silent touching of Jesus' clothes is preceded by her trust that if this can be done 'I shall be made well' (Mark 5.28 / Matt. 9.21).

In a number of stories faithful trust in Jesus as healer takes the form of verbal persistence rather than determined silent action. It is this which Jesus appeared to commend in Mark's story of blind Bartimaeus and in Luke's parallel story (Mark 10.52 / Luke 18.42); in Matthew and Luke's story of the centurion and his servant (Matt. 8.10 / Luke 7.9), albeit in Luke's version this is heightened by the centurion using his friends to relay his messages to Jesus; and in Matthew's version of the Canaanite woman (15.28). In the last two stories the non-Jewish origins of those begging for healing enhances both their persistence and the subsequent commendation of their faith.

There is one particular story where *pistis* understood as 'faithful trust in Jesus as healer' becomes explicit, namely Matthew's story of the two blind men. After their initial persistence:

Jesus said to them, 'Do you believe [*pisteuete*] that I am able to do this?' They said to him, 'Yes, Lord.' Then he touched their eyes, saying, 'According to your faith [*pistin*] be it done to you.' And their eyes were opened. (Matt. 9.28b–30a)

So the 'faith' of the two blind men here seems to have been simply 'that I am able to do this'. Once they had demonstrated this faith – perhaps both by their initial persistence and by their actual assent to Jesus' direct question – then healing followed. Is that all that 'faith' denotes in the Synoptic healing stories?

Mark's account of the healing of the epileptic boy might suggest as much until, that is, the mention of prayer in the final verse. There was an initial failure of the disciples to heal the boy; Jesus' response about a faithless generation; the account of the illness by the boy's father with a request to have pity 'if you can do anything'; Jesus' response about all things being possible 'to him who believes'; the father's cry of faith; and then the healing. All of this fits a similar pattern of the 'faith' required being simply 'that I am able to do this'. But then (in Mark alone) the disciples asked Jesus why they had been unable to cast out the boy's unclean spirit and Jesus responded that, 'This kind cannot be driven out by anything but prayer' (9.29). Faith is now set at a quite different level – that is, as response to God.[44] Similarly the story of the paralytic man, in all three Gospels here, concludes with the crowd giving glory to God for the healing. Luke also has the man himself giving glory to God separately (5.25) and Matthew adds significantly that, 'they glorified God, who had given such authority to men' (9.7). When it is also recalled how often healing stories in Mark are associated with Jesus teaching in a synagogue, it is clear that *pistis* within the assumptions of the Synoptic healing stories cannot be limited simply to the mundane trust that someone is able to effect a healing. It *is* that, but it is also clearly more than that: beyond the mundane, faith, properly understood, is response to God.

'Faith' in both of these senses – faith as trust in the healer and faith as response to God – will be explored in relation to modern health care ethics in chapter 6. However there is also a third sense, based upon mutuality, which is present in some of the stories. It seems to be present in Luke's puzzling story of the ten lepers. C. F. Evans points out the problem with this particular story ending with the formula 'your faith has made you well':

Elsewhere this either effects the healing or accompanies it (cf. 8.48; 18.42 and the parallels in Mark), but here it comes belatedly as a comment on it, and as

---

[44] Cf. Marshall, *Faith*, pp. 221–3.

a somewhat conventional rounding off of the story as a miracle story. For Luke cannot have meant that only the Samaritan was healed by faith, the rest being healed without faith. The sharp point for which the story is told, and which cannot be made without it, is Jesus' commendation, not of faith as such, nor of thanksgiving in general, but of the genuine piety of a non-Israelite manifesting itself in gratitude.[45]

In Luke's story the other nine lepers apparently did show faith, both in appealing to Jesus for mercy in the first place and then in obeying his command to go and show themselves to the priests. Although they were healed, they did not reciprocate with either praise to God or prostrate gratitude to Jesus (and therefore, so more conservative scholars than Evans tend to argue, they were not actually 'saved';[46] Malina, in contrast, argues that to 'thank Jesus would mean that the relationship is over').[47] There was healing but little mutuality. And in one incident in Mark and Matthew, despite being set in a synagogue, there was apparently such an absence of faith/mutuality that there was little healing at all (Mark 6.5 / Matt. 13.58). A full account of faith in the Synoptic healing stories needs to add mutuality to the two other levels of trust in the healer and response to God.

HUMILITY

The fourth and concluding feature of the healing stories is a command for restraint. How is this to be understood in a context of healing? It is surprising how little attention is given to this question in biblical commentaries. The basic problem seems to be that, despite a widespread agreement that it does not actually work, many commentators still feel obliged to focus upon Wrede's theory of the so-called messianic secret when considering commands to silence within the Synoptic healing stories.

Writing fifty years ago, even then Vincent Taylor admitted that 'in the form in which Wrede presented it, the theory has been widely rejected, but it continues to exert a great influence . . . the citadel has

---

[45] Evans, *Saint Luke*, p. 623.
[46] E.g. I. Howard Marshall, *The Gospel of Luke* (Exeter: Paternoster, 1978), pp. 648–9.
[47] Malina, *The New Testament World*, p. 93.

caved in; but the flag still flies'.[48] For Wrede the commands to silence were an unhistorical device of the early church to explain why Jesus was not recognised as the Messiah during his life-time. In Taylor's revised form the theory becomes an expression of Jesus' own conception of Messiahship: knowing himself to be already the Messiah, not least through his healings, he nonetheless commanded silence until his destiny was fulfilled after the Resurrection. Yet even in this modified form this theory hardly fits the exceptions to silence already noted (Mark 5.19 / Luke 8.39, Matt. 11.4–5 / Luke 7.22 and Luke 13.32).

Another four decades later, Morna Hooker's discussion of the commands to silence is still dominated by Wrede. She rejects Taylor's revised theory and agrees with Wrede that the commands are (largely) an unhistorical device. However, she differs from Wrede in her interpretation of the function of this device:

It seems clear the commands to secrecy are largely (though not necessarily entirely) artificial, and that they are a narrative device which has been used by Mark to draw his reader's attention to the real significance of his story. Secrecy and disclosure are part of a theme which pervades the whole of Mark's gospel. Throughout the narrative, Jesus acts with supreme authority yet makes no open claims for himself ... Yet for those with eyes and ears to see and hear, the meaning is plain ... The truth about Jesus is at once hidden from view and yet spelt out on every page of the gospel.[49]

It is only at this point in her discussion that Hooker suggests that there may be another plausible explanation of the commands. She regards it as an open question whether Mark created these commands entirely himself or whether some might actually have come from an earlier tradition reflecting Jesus' own ministry (interestingly, and in sharp contrast, the form critic Gerd Theissen concluded that 'probably all the commands to silence in miracle stories are from the tradition').[50] However, on the supposition that some of commands may not be Mark's own creations, she suggests:

If we believe that Jesus' actions were characterized by an authority which may fairly be termed 'messianic', then it is possible that the so-called

---

[48] Taylor, *The Gospel According to St Mark*, pp. 122–3.
[49] Hooker, *The Gospel According to St Mark*, pp. 68–9.   [50] Theissen, *Miracle Stories*, p. 150.

messianic secret reflects not simply the tension between Jesus as he was perceived in his lifetime and as he was confessed after the resurrection, but the reluctance of Jesus to make claims about himself: for his message was centred on God and on his Kingdom, not on himself, and if he believed himself to be in any sense the Messiah, the last thing he would do was to claim the title for himself.[51]

In other words, reticence may have been an expression of humility.

Once Wrede's theory is no longer allowed to dominate interpretations of the commands to silence, it is possible that this final suggestion may actually be more fruitful in the specific context of healing. Within this context there are some very obvious and pressing reasons for taking humility seriously. Public and personalised claims to have special powers of healing – although often made by crusading faith healers – are notoriously treacherous. Unless they are to resort to chicanery, mundane faith healers soon find them impossible to fulfil. Even Jesus within the Synoptic Gospels, as just noted, was unable to heal many in a context that lacked faith/mutuality. Worse still, such claims soon attract unwelcome crowd expectations, both within the ancient world and, rather oddly, within modern pluralistic societies. Crowd elation, hysteria, recriminations, exaggerated claims and polemical counter-claims are soon made. In short, an absence of restraint in this area soon leads to a serious loss of control. In chapter 7 it will be argued that this can be so even in modern, conventional forms of medicine. Humility has an important role to play in modern health care ethics.

A pattern of reticence in a context of exaggerated crowd expectations can soon be detected in the Synoptic Gospels. The threatening role of the crowd in the early chapters of Mark has already been noted. Yet it is also a feature of Matthew. In their commentary on Matthew, Davies and Allison appear to agree with Wrede's conclusion that 'the idea of the messianic secret no longer has the importance for Matthew that it has for Mark'.[52] They note, for example, that Matthew drops six of Mark's commands to silence. However this conclusion fails to observe the overall pattern of, say, chapters 8 and 9

---

[51] Hooker, *The Gospel According to St Mark*, p. 69.
[52] Davies and Allison, *A Critical Commentary on The Gospel According to Saint Matthew*, vol. II, p. 14.

in Matthew. Although two of Mark's commands are dropped here, another is introduced from Matthew's own source and then placed in a strategic point in the narrative. An overall pattern of reticence, movement and troubled crowds emerges: Jesus comes down from the mountain and great crowds follow him (8.1); Jesus commands the leper to silence (8.4); Jesus enters Capernaum (8.5); Jesus sees great crowds surrounding him and gives orders to get away (8.18); Jesus crosses over by boat to the country of the Gadarenes (8.28); all the city come out to meet Jesus and beg him to leave (8.34); Jesus crosses back by boat (9.1); the crowds see the healing of the paralytic and are afraid (9.8); Jesus puts the crowd outside before raising the ruler's daughter (9.25); Jesus sternly commands the two blind men to silence (9.30); crowds are moved at the healing of the dumb demoniac (9.33); but the Pharisees make hostile counter-claims (9.34); Jesus goes about cities and villages preaching and healing (9.35); Jesus has compassion for the crowds (9.36).

Reticence following exaggerated crowd expectations might also be detected in the later traditions of healing stories to be found in John and Acts. Earlier commentators tended to make much of the contrast between Mark and these later sources, since the latter lack explicit commands to silence either by Jesus (in John) or by the apostles (in Acts). Both of these later sources also make much about healings as 'signs' (e.g. John 4.54 and Acts 4.16: in this Acts context Peter even preaches two sermons on the strength of a single healing). Yet, viewed from the specific perspective of healing: Jesus apparently withdrew because of the crowd after healing a sick man at the pool (John 5.13); he could no longer go 'about among the Jews' after raising Lazarus (John 11.54); 'jealousy' against the apostles was prompted by crowds being healed by them (Acts 5.12–18); and Peter put all the weeping women outside before healing a woman at Joppa (Acts 9.40).

Of course such reticence in a context of exaggerated crowd expectations can never be absolute. Despite being sternly commanded to silence by Jesus, Matthew recounts that the two blind men 'went away and spread his fame through all that district' (9.31). And, away from pressing crowds, the exceptions to commands to silence even in the earliest Gospel traditions no longer appear so odd. It is precisely within a context of exaggerated crowd expectations that the boastful claims of ancient or modern faith healers become so damaging.

In contrast, the healer who is really concerned to heal will be much more humble and cautious about public claims.

Humility, compassion, care and faith are all virtues expressed in many religious traditions. In the chapters that follow, I will argue that they also have a distinctive and important contribution to make to health care ethics today even within the public forum of a Western, pluralistic society.

CHAPTER 4

Compassion in health care ethics

Compassion offers a double critique: of much secular health care ethics for not making compassion sufficiently explicit and of a number of Christian versions of health care ethics for failing to place compassion before even principled scruples. Compassion, properly understood, is an essential starting point for health care ethics even within a pluralistic society. Within the Synoptic healing stories compassion is not simply about feeling sorry for the vulnerable, nor is it even just about empathy, a preparedness to identify with the vulnerable. Rather, compassion is both a response to the vulnerable and a determination to help them, sometimes at the expense of principled scruples.

Oliver Davies' powerful book *A Theology of Compassion* makes a sustained case for regarding compassion as the primary Christian virtue. His concern is with theology as a whole rather than with the specific area of healing. Nevertheless what he writes can easily be applied to the latter. He argues that compassion rather than love best depicts the Christian life, since love 'embraces concepts and phenomena that are both wholly distinct and easily confused' (such as *agape* and *eros*):

Compassion, on the other hand, presents a complex but more easily identifiable structure, which in Martha Nussbaum's analysis entails a combination of cognitive, affective and volitional elements. In compassion we see another's distress (cognition), we feel moved by it (affectively) and we actively seek to remedy it (volition).[1]

This combination of cognitive, affective and volitional elements is exactly what characterises mercy/compassion in the Synoptic healing stories. At the outset Jesus is made aware of those in serious need

---

[1] Oliver Davies, *A Theology of Compassion* (London: SCM Press, 2001), pp. 17–18.

explicitly or implicitly begging him for mercy (cognition). He responds by stopping, listening, talking and showing anger/compassion (affectively). He then acts, touching even those who are regarded as ritually unclean, cleansing and healing them (volition). Empathy can remain largely at the cognitive level and sympathy at the affective level. However, compassion, properly understood, involves cognitive, affective *and* volitional elements. The one who is properly compassionate seeks, wherever possible, to remedy another's distress.

Davies recognises, of course, that for ordinary mortals there is not always a remedy:

That man or woman who understands another's suffering and is affected by it, while recognising that action on behalf of that person is simply not possible (as in the case of terminal illness for instance), can be said to be compassionate, since it is simply practical constraints which prevent the expression of the will to alleviate suffering.[2]

The Synoptic Gospel writers would have recognised no such practical constraints confronting Jesus. However, in the more mundane context of health care ethics today it is crucial. Volition is an essential element of compassion even when it is finally thwarted by human limitations.

Another helpful point that Davies makes is that compassion is not an exclusively Judaeo-Christian concept. It is both an essential civil virtue and a requirement of many religious traditions:

Compassion stands at the far end of a continuum of altruistic actions, which begins in the domain of everyday experience. Indeed, a good deal of human behaviour can only be explained by reference to an altruism which is not the refined calculation of self-interest. The principle of self-denying or kenotic love, of which compassion is a particularly radical manifestation, appears to touch all levels of human existence and, indeed, to make harmonious existence possible. Without such a principle of self-emptying for the sake of the other, enacted in some degree by a myriad of people in countless different ways, most human societies could not keep at bay the violent and selfish tendencies of the human spirit ... Despite all the ambiguities of human motivation and understanding, and the social, cultural and psychological complexities of human interaction, such acts of exceptional self-giving love appear to many to represent a moral ideal and to reflect in

---

[2] Davies, *A Theology of Compassion*, p. 18.

radical form a principle of altruism without which social civilization as such would founder. It is also significant in this respect that the major world religions combine in laying a particular stress upon the place of compassion in the hierarchy of spiritual values.[3]

In a footnote at the end of this paragraph he refers specifically to the concept of *karunā* in Buddhism, 'humaneness' in the Confucian tradition, and *rahmah* in Islam.[4] Indeed, even a superficial reading of the Qu'ran soon confirms the centrality of compassion within Islam. Every *sura* (or chapter) but one begins with the invocation 'In the Name of God, the Merciful, the Compassionate'. There are frequent reminders to the faithful in the Qu'ran that they should in turn be compassionate to the poor, the needy and travellers (e.g. XXX.35) and followers of Jesus are commended because 'We set in the hearts of those who followed him tenderness and mercy' (LVII.25).[5]

One of the features of compassion within the Synoptic Gospels that Davies tends to overlook is the way it can trump principled scruples. In a Jewish context of principled scruples about the impurity of disease and disability, the Synoptic Jesus is repeatedly moved by compassion, or by pleas for mercy, to touch (or to allow himself to be touched by) those deemed to be impure. Matthew expresses this succinctly in his story of the two blind men at Jericho:

Moved with compassion [*splagxnistheis*], Jesus touched their eyes. (Matt. 20.34)

This pattern regularly punctuates the first half of Mark (even the disputed variant reading of 'pity' in the first of the following quotations does not destroy this pattern since the leper is already depicted as 'begging'):

A leper came to him begging him, and kneeling said to him, 'If you choose, you can make me clean.' Moved with pity, Jesus stretched out his hand and touched him, and said to him, 'I do choose. Be made clean!' (Mark 1.40–1)

---

[3] Davies, *A Theology of Compassion*, pp. 20–1.

[4] See further, Peter Harvey, *An Introduction to Buddhism* (Cambridge: Cambridge University Press, 1990), pp. 209–12; Xinzhong Yao, *An Introduction to Confucianism* (Cambridge: Cambridge University Press, 2000); and Kenneth Cragg, *The Mind of the Qu'ran* (London: Allen & Unwin, 1973), pp. 110–28.

[5] The translation of the Qu'ran used is Arthur J. Arberry, *The Koran Interpreted* (Oxford: Oxford University Press, 1998).

Then one of the leaders of the synagogue named Jairus came and, when he saw him, fell at his feet and begged him repeatedly, 'My little daughter is at the point of death. Come and lay your hands on her.' (Mark 5.22–3)

And wherever he went, into villages or cities or farms, they laid the sick in the marketplaces, and begged him that they might touch even the fringe of his cloak; and all who touched it were healed. (Mark 6.56)

They brought to him a deaf man who had an impediment in his speech; and they begged him to lay his hand on him. He took him aside in private, away from the crowd, and put his fingers into his ears, and he spat and touched his tongue. (Mark 7.32–3)

Some people brought a blind man to him and begged him to touch him. (Mark 8.22)

Jesus asked the father. 'How long has this been happening to him?' And he said, 'From childhood. It has often cast him into the fire and into the water, to destroy him; but if you are able to do anything, have pity on us and help us' . . . Jesus took him by the hand and lifted him up. (Mark 9.21–2 and 27)

To these instances can be added the tendency of Mark to set healing stories on the Sabbath.

Biblical scholars continue to debate whether Jesus was an observant Jew who nevertheless rejected the Pharisees' excessive notions of ritual purity or a Jew concerned to challenge ritual purity more radically.[6] Whichever is finally judged to be more apposite, there is a repeated pattern here of the Synoptic Jesus allowing compassion to trump principled scruples (whether these scruples are his own or those of others). Marcus Borg depicts this as an ambivalent clash between two codes, a holiness/purity code on the one hand and a compassion code on the other. Jesus advocated 'replacing holiness with compassion as the core value of Israel's life' and 'consistently, "compassion" appears in opposition to holiness or to behavior mandated by holiness':[7] For Borg, 'contrary to the "holiness code" which undergirded resistance, the "compassion code" urged love of enemies and the way of peace . . . the "compassion code" strikes

---

[6] See James D. G. Dunn, 'Jesus and Purity: an Ongoing Debate', *New Testament Studies*, 48 (2002), pp. 449–67.

[7] Marcus J. Borg, *Conflict, Holiness and Politics in the Teaching of Jesus* (Harrisburg, PA: Trinity Press International, 2nd edn, 1998), p. 135.

a new but complementary note'.[8] Yet, paradoxically, Jesus still taught 'holiness', albeit holiness now 'understood as a transforming power, not as a power that needed protection through rigorous separation'.[9]

The story of the healing of Simon's mother-in-law may involve a double infringement of principled scruples or old-style 'holiness codes' (i.e. healing on the Sabbath and touching a diseased person):

As soon as they left the synagogue, they entered the house of Simon and Andrew, with James and John. Now Simon's mother-in-law was in bed with a fever, and they told him about her at once. He came and took her by the hand and lifted her up. (Mark 1.29–31)

Luke's unique story of the healing of a crippled woman may also illustrate the same theme of compassion trumping principled scruples. The woman's condition is depicted in a way perhaps intended by Luke to evoke compassion:

And just then there appeared a woman with a spirit that had crippled her for eighteen years. She was bent over, and was quite unable to stand up straight. (Luke 13.11–12)

Despite being in a synagogue on the Sabbath, Jesus called her over and laid his hands upon her. The principled scruples of the leader of the synagogue in this story are entirely logical (would another day really have mattered?):

There are six days on which work ought to be done; come on those days and be cured, and not on the Sabbath day. (Luke 13.14b)

In response, Jesus put his opponents 'to shame' by reminding them that even they act (compassionately) to their animals on the Sabbath. Christopher Evans points out that, in contrast:

The Qumran community appears to have been more rigorous in ordering that 'no man shall assist a beast to give birth on the Sabbath day. And if it shall fall into a cistern or pit, he shall not lift it out on the Sabbath.'[10]

---

[8] Borg, *Conflict*, p. 145.   [9] Borg, *Conflict*, p. 147.
[10] C. F. Evans, *Saint Luke* (London and Philadelphia: SCM Press and Trinity Press, 1990), p. 551.

IMPLICIT COMPASSION

Within secular health care ethics an explicit attention to the role of compassion might help to narrow the moral gap between personal resonance and a shared understanding of cosmic order. Even within a pluralistic society there may in reality be more common ground on compassion than is sometimes supposed. It is notoriously difficult to find agreement on common goods within a pluralistic society (as critics of natural law have often maintained), but it may be somewhat easier to agree upon common ills.

In his contribution to New Studies in Christian Ethics Gordon Graham argues that there is more implicit agreement today about what is wrong, or even evil, than is generally recognised.[11] For example, he suggests that across different religious and secular traditions around the world there is now common agreement that human slavery is wrong. Of course he is aware that it was sometimes justified in the past and tragically that it is still practised illegally today (perhaps even in Britain). Yet, he argues, a significant difference between the past and present is that even those who perpetuate human slavery today do not claim that it is morally justified. Both perpetrators and abolitionists today *know* that human slavery is wrong. In a similar vein, Graham explores the horrific world of the serial killer, showing in the process that, although such killing can become disturbingly seductive to the perpetrator, he (it usually is a 'he') typically becomes only gradually desensitised to its evilness. Graham writes as a professional philosopher and as a Christian, so he is concerned to demonstrate that evil is an objective reality and not simply a human creation, let alone a product of changing and changeable human tastes.

Writing from a non-religious perspective, the bioethicist Jonathan Glover's major work *Humanity: a Moral History of the Twentieth Century* does see ethics (and presumably evil) purely as a human creation. He writes in considerable, and frequently moving, detail about some of the major human 'atrocities' enacted over the last hundred years. He is conscious that in previous centuries war, tribalism and terror have disfigured humanity, but that modern technology has exacerbated the scale of these atrocities in the twentieth

---

[11] Gordon Graham, *Evil and Christian Ethics* (Cambridge: Cambridge University Press, 2001).

century. He charts at length atrocities such as the trenches of the First
World War, the systematic terrors of Stalin, Hitler and Mao, and
then Hiroshima, My Lai and Rwanda. At every point he seeks to
understand how human beings can do such terrible things to other
human beings. In part his aim is 'to replace the thin, mechanical
psychology of the Enlightenment with something more complex,
something closer to reality':[12]

At the start of the century there was an optimism, coming from the
Enlightenment, that the spread of a humane and scientific outlook would
lead to the fading away, not only of war, but also of other forms of cruelty
and barbarism. They would fill the chamber of horrors in the museum of
our primitive past. In the light of these expectations, the century of Hitler,
Stalin, Pol Pot and Saddam Hussein was likely to be a surprise. Volcanoes
thought extinct turned out not to be.[13]

At every point in the book Glover's bleak reading of post-
Enlightenment human action is accompanied by both a strong sense
of moral outrage (he frequently uses the word 'atrocity') and an
obvious sense of compassion. Yet there is also wistfulness in the book
and it is not entirely clear how he finally grounds either the moral
outrage or the compassion in a convincing secular, moral philosophy:

One of the features of our time is the fading of the moral law. The idea of a
moral law external to us may never have had secure foundations, but, partly
because of the decline of religion in the Western world, awareness of this is
now widespread. Those of us who do not believe in a religious moral law
should still be troubled by its fading. The evils of religious intolerance,
religious persecution and religious wars are well known, but it is striking
how many protests against and acts of resistance to atrocity have also come
from principled religious commitment . . . The decline of this moral commitment would be a huge loss.[14]

He is conscious that some will regard his own secular solution as
'vague', but finally all that he can offer is that:

As authority-based morality retreats, it can be replaced by a morality which
is deliberately created. The best hope is to work with the grain of human

[12] Jonathan Glover, *Humanity: a Moral History of the Twentieth Century* (London: Jonathan
Cape, 1999), p. 7.
[13] Glover, *Humanity*, p. 6.   [14] Glover, *Humanity*, p. 405.

nature, making use of the resources of moral identity and the human responses.[15]

The difficulty for a Christian ethicist at this point is even to imagine how a morality 'which is deliberately created' will ever be remotely convincing, let alone how it can avoid the bleak atrocities that Glover has so convincingly shown to be a substantial part of 'human nature'. It is surely ironic that Hitler, Stalin, and Pol Pot (and perhaps even Saddam Hussein), as determined secularists, did indeed attempt to promote moralities that were 'deliberately created', not least to enhance their power over their own people. The immense achievement of *Humanity: a Moral History of the Twentieth Century* is to depict so frankly and compassionately the scale of human atrocity that characterised the twentieth century. Its failure is to ground it in a wistful hope for 'a morality which is deliberately created'.

To set this into Glover's more familiar area of health care ethics, it could be that even if people cannot agree about what constitutes 'well being', most might agree about what generally constitutes illness or disability and that, other things being equal, it is desirable to find ways of reducing or eliminating them. Of course there will still be some areas where agreement remains elusive – for example, whether deafness constitutes a disability within signing families – but these areas are vastly outnumbered even within a Western, pluralistic society by areas of general agreement. And meta-ethical differences will remain about whether this agreement is entirely the result of cultural determinants or whether it is based, at least in part, in human nature (as natural law theorists hold, albeit with very different internal balances).[16] Yet there may still be general agreement that it is desirable to reduce or eliminate illness and disability. Here there does seem, even within a pluralistic society, to be a level of agreement that goes beyond personal resonance or arbitrary creation.

Compassion as a virtue is, however, more than a general agreement that it is desirable to reduce or eliminate illness and disability. It is both a response to the ill and disabled and a determination to help them.

---

[15] Glover, *Humanity*, p. 409.
[16] See Stephen J. Pope, 'Natural Law and Christian Ethics', in Robin Gill (ed.), *The Cambridge Companion to Christian Ethics* (Cambridge: Cambridge University Press, 2001).

It is this starting point in compassion that is so obviously missing from the four principles approach to health care ethics (autonomy, non-maleficence, beneficence and justice) discussed earlier in chapter 1. The four principles are, to apply an analogy, more akin to principles governing *ius in bello* than *ius ad bellum*. That is to say, they suggest criteria to be considered carefully within the context of medical intervention, but they do not denote what drives, motivates, deepens and embeds that intervention. In their careful critique of Beauchamp and Childress (and also of Engelhardt's variation of the four principles approach),[17] Scott Rae and Paul Cox make this point effectively:

What may be more important than giving health care workers a set of principles is teaching them to be the kind of persons they must be to properly function in the health care arena. Moreover, health care workers need to remember the goal or end of medicine more than they need principles by which to solve supposed ethical dilemmas. Most of the questions, issues, and dilemmas raised in the medical arena can be resolved by reminding health care workers of the aim of their work as well as helping them develop the appropriate character traits that undergird and facilitate that end. While Beauchamp and Childress indicate an awareness that character is important, their focus on principles prevents them from according it adequate weight. For Beauchamp and Childress, the relationship between, say, the physician and the patient is primarily contractual. The duties of this contractual relationship flow from the 'principles of bioethical ethics' rather than from the nature of the activity of care and healing.[18]

There is even a developing consensus among a number of Christian and secular bioethicists that the four principles approach of Beauchamp and Childress is not so much wrong as just 'thin'. So, the philosopher Onora O'Neill[19] argues at length that their concept of 'autonomy' needs to be made considerably thicker using a Kantian concept of 'principled autonomy' (chapter 6 will return to this). And there is a surprising level of similar agreement among the religious

---

[17] See H. Tristram Engelhardt Jr, *The Foundations of Bioethics* (New York: Oxford University Press, 2nd edn, 1996).

[18] Scott B. Rae and Paul M. Cox (eds.), *Bioethics: a Christian Approach in a Pluralistic Age* (Grand Rapids, MI: William B. Eerdmans, 1999), p. 78.

[19] Onora O'Neill, *Autonomy and Trust in Bioethics* (Cambridge: Cambridge University Press, 2002). See also Gordon M. Stirrat and Robin Gill, 'Autonomy in Medical Ethics after O'Neill', *Journal of Medical Ethics*, 31:2 (2005), pp. 127–30.

and non-religious bioethicists contributing to the edition of the *Journal of Medical Ethics* marking Raanan Gillon's retirement after two decades as editor. In this Gillon challenges others to evaluate the four principles approach in the light of specified case studies in health care ethics. Daniel Callahan, veteran of the Hastings Centre, concludes that this approach, despite its congeniality in a 'liberal, individualistic culture' and its relative simplicity within clinical decision-making, is finally 'too narrow to do all the necessary work of ethics, too individualistic to help answer the questions about the appropriate needs of communities, and too mechanical to encourage some necessary analytical and personal skills'.[20] Alastair Campbell, bioethicist and pastoral theologian, agrees that this approach is too thin on its own and argues that a combination of virtue ethics and the four principles is needed instead:

I conclude that virtue ethics and the four principles are 'partners in crime' when it comes to the final justification of our moral intuitions. Each captures different dimensions of our moral universe, but one is not better than the other in settling finally how we make correct moral judgments. The principles help us to structure our reasoning when faced with novel moral challenges and they remind us of key questions to be explored. Virtue ethics directs us to the character of the decision maker, but also to the implications for our whole lives and for society of individual choices and policy decisions.[21]

There are some remaining differences between Campbell and the non-religious bioethicist Raanan Gillon, but their final positions are remarkably close. So Gillon expresses his own as follows:

Virtues – morally desirable dispositions of character – are needed both for moral obligations to be instantiated and sustained in the moral life of real people and for all sorts of other supererogatory but morally desirable aspects of life. In relation to universalisable moral obligations, moral principles – or at least some moral norms, standards or values – are needed to decide *which* dispositions of character are to be properly regarded as virtuous and in which circumstances, which vicious, and which neither the one nor the other.[22]

---

[20] D. Callahan, 'Principlism and Communitarianism', *Journal of Medical Ethics*, 29:5 (2003), p. 291.

[21] A. V. Campbell, 'The Virtues (and Vices) of the Four Principles', *Journal of Medical Ethics*, 29:5 (2003), p. 293.

[22] R. Gillon, 'Ethics Needs Principles – four can encompass the rest – and respect for autonomy should be "first among equals"', *Journal of Medical Ethics*, 29:5 (2003), p. 309.

My own position is finally closer to that of Campbell. A combination of virtue ethics (drawing virtues explicitly from the Synoptic healing stories – involving both individual character and a conception of the common good) and the four principles (in order to structure and prompt moral reasoning) is axiomatic to this book. It is even possible that such an approach might be able to appeal to theological realists such as Campbell and myself as well as to theological purists such as Gilbert Meilaender. It is surely instructive that the latter argues as follows:

> Ultimately, however, it is more important to see that the theory is 'thin' than that it is sometimes idle. *Principles of Biomedical Ethics* often fails to provide the kind of wisdom we need most. Beauchamp and Childress acknowledge that application of their principles will 'depend on factual beliefs about the world'.[23] How we describe a situation will depend on the background beliefs – scientific, metaphysical, and religious – that we bring to it. They recognize the relevance of such beliefs but are seldom willing to explore them in detail.[24]

Perhaps it is not so much that compassion is missing from such 'thin' approaches to health care ethics but rather that it is too implicit rather than explicit. So, from time to time the word 'compassion' does occur in the British Medical Association's *Medical Ethics Today*[25] and there is even an acknowledgement within it that BMA research has confirmed that 'compassion' is one of the core values of British doctors. Nevertheless, it is still principles such as autonomy, non-maleficence, beneficence and justice that predominate in this core guidance for doctors.

A focus upon compassion also offers a critique of a number of positions in Christian ethics, especially those engaged with 'status of life' issues. All too often Christian (as well as Orthodox Jewish and Muslim) interventions in the public forum on these issues appear to

[23] Tom L. Beauchamp and James F. Childress, *Principles of Biomedical Ethics* (Oxford and New York: Oxford University Press, 4th edn, 1994), p. 7.

[24] Gilbert Meilaender, *Body, Soul and Bioethics* (Notre Dame, IN: University of Notre Dame Press, 1995), p. 15. For a similar Catholic critique, see Benedict M. Ashley and Kevin D. O'Rourke, *Health Care and Ethics: a Theological Analysis* (Washington, DC: Georgetown University Press, 4th edn, 1996), pp. 221–2.

[25] British Medical Association Ethics Department, *Medical Ethics Today* (London: BMJ Books, 2004).

have been more concerned with maintaining principled scruples than with starting (like the Synoptic Jesus) from compassion. Although a commitment to compassion does not in itself resolve dilemmas in health care ethics, it does suggest priorities.

Lisa Cahill's warning, cited in chapter 1, is again important: 'the prevailing discourse has managed virtually to equate "religious bioethics" with such advocacy, constructing it as a public danger, even while insisting on its marginality ... religion is framed as entirely preoccupied with "status of life" issues'.[26] John Hinnells and Roy Porter, in the introduction to their unique symposium *Religion, Health and Suffering*, offer an even starker warning:

The interaction between religion and medicine is universal throughout recorded history. They meet at the great turning points of life: at birth, at moments of acute suffering and at death. Not only are priest and doctor often needed at the same time and place, the two roles have also been combined in ancient and modern societies ... However, relations between healers and religious leaders have not always been good. In modern Western society established churches, both Catholic and Evangelical, have objected, indeed obstructed, some surgical procedures such as abortion. Similarly in the nineteenth century, many Christians objected to the medical alleviation of pain in childbirth ... It should also be said that many religious leaders in religions the world over, have inflicted suffering and torture in order to obtain converts or punish heretics. Religions have not always been the caring forces their adherents sometimes emphasise![27]

Abortion certainly remains a major religious fault-line in the modern world, as well as being a fault-line within world religions themselves.[28] For some religious ethicists principled scruples about when meaningful human life begins should give way to compassion for women faced with burdensome pregnancies in an already over-populated world – or indeed for embryonic stem cell research seeking

---

[26] Lisa Sowle Cahill, 'Bioethics, Theology, and Social Change', *Journal of Religious Ethics*, 31:3 (2003), p. 371.

[27] John R. Hinnells and Roy Porter (eds.), *Religion, Health and Suffering* (London and New York: Kegan Paul International, 1999), p. xi. See also Ronald L. Numbers and Darrel W. Amundsen (eds.), *Caring and Curing: Health and Medicine in the Western Religious Traditions* (London and New York: Macmillan, 1986).

[28] See Daniel C. Maguire, *Sacred Choices: the Right to Contraception and Abortion in Ten World Religions* (Minneapolis: Fortress Press, 2001).

cures for serious genetic conditions. For others such a position is ethically and theologically objectionable.[29]

Andrzej Kulczycki[30] provides an instructive account of current abortion practice and politics in three contrasting countries – Kenya, Mexico and Poland – in which the Catholic Church is strong and influential. In Kenya three-quarters of the population is Christian, with the Catholic Church being the largest denomination. The average size of families there is declining rapidly and there is a growing use of legal and illegal abortions. He sets out how the Kenyan Catholic bishops have argued consistently against abortion itself and also against sex education in schools and the issue of condoms to prevent HIV/AIDS (chapter 5 will return to this last issue). In the face of growing problems in Kenya, and elsewhere in Africa today, Kulczycki depicts the situation as 'a tyranny of silence'. Most people in Mexico and Poland are, at least nominally, Catholic and Pope John Paul II used his visits there to condemn what he termed the 'culture of death' that promotes contraception and abortion. However, in Mexico a long tradition of revolutionary politics and anti-clericalism have existed alongside popular cultural Catholicism. The result, Kulczycki argues, is some of the most restrictive abortion laws in the world. Yet illegal abortions, and septic deaths resulting from them, are common. In contrast, the communist authorities in Poland introduced a very liberal abortion law in 1956, which, in the absence of effective contraceptives, resulted in high (but relatively safe) abortion rates, even among churchgoers. Kulczycki suggests that, ironically, in Poland and Mexico 'some Catholic women have more qualms about using contraception than resorting to abortion, owing to a peculiar interpretation of a Catholic rationalism ... a woman confessing to an abortion has only to request a pardon once and she is forgiven, whereas she would be repeatedly sinning if she used contraception'.[31] The bishops in Poland have since liberation in 1989 systematically attempted to overturn the liberal abortion law. Their efforts were at first successful, but then provoked

---

[29] See Edmund D. Pellegrino and Alan I. Faden (eds.), *Jewish and Catholic Bioethics: an Ecumenical Dialogue* (Washington, DC: Georgetown University Press, 1999), pp. 15–74.

[30] Andrzej Kulczycki, *The Abortion Debate in the World Arena* (London: Macmillan, 1999).

[31] Kulczycki, *Abortion Debate*, p. 96.

a serious political backlash. Kulczycki believes that, as a result, the church has lost considerable influence in Poland today and even provoked anti-clericalism despite its previous popularity.

As a specialist in population studies Kulczycki is more concerned to assess the social and political consequences of this Catholic opposition to abortion than to evaluate its theological merits. He identifies two in particular. The first of these is as follows:

The Church will always speak out on moral and social issues, but the abortion debate raises age-old questions about the reasonable limits of the Church's involvement (or that of other religious bodies) in the public sphere. It highlights the difficulties of remaining faithful to an ethical position while attempting to develop a public policy that is legislatively feasible. In Catholic countries it also brings up the vexing question of whether the law should mirror the Church's social teachings, as in Ireland or Poland (1993–96), or less directly reflect them, as in Belgium, France, Spain, Portugal or Italy.[32]

His second point is closer to that of Lisa Cahill:

In seeking to make abortion a binding moral concern for all Catholics, the rest of the Church's social teaching is downplayed both in the Church's priority of concerns and in the eyes of politicians and the public. In the USA this has prevented the Catholic Church (the largest private health care provider in the country) from lending its considerable weight to supporting the cause of universal health care coverage, a long cherished goal.[33]

How far should religious people go to oppose abortion? This question is particularly important for those who are convinced that, to put it bluntly, induced abortion is murder. Since 1869 (and, according to David Albert Jones, for very much longer)[34] the Vatican has argued that from the moment of conception the embryo is a full human being with a soul that survives death – not simply a potential human being – and should always be treated as such. Those who agree with this position face a very serious problem. If individuals wish, say, to commit adultery, then however much others might disapprove, few in the West today would think it right to punish them by law (although of course people have in the past).

---

[32] Kulczycki, *Abortion Debate*, p. 159.   [33] Kulczycki, *Abortion Debate*, p. 162.
[34] David Albert Jones, *The Soul of the Embryo: an Enquiry into the Status of the Human Embryo in the Christian Tradition* (London: Continuum, 2004).

But what about murder? We usually do everything in our power to stop that. So if abortion (including forms of contraception which prevent implantation and embryonic stem cell research) is murder, surely we should do the same? Given this logic, it is obvious why the abortion/contraception issue above all else has politicised previously a-political Catholics so strongly in many countries.

The journalists James Risen and Judy L. Thomas in *Wrath of Angels: the American Abortion War*[35] give a deeply disturbing, even if anecdotal, account of a third social consequence of 'Christian' opposition to abortion. They trace the events leading up to the religiously motivated murder of several people involved in abortion clinics. In the early 1970s a charismatic Catholic layperson, John O'Keefe, started to organise peaceful opposition to abortion clinics. Yet he soon began to attract more violent Christian followers, such as Michael Bray. Pickets and banners were regularly paraded outside abortion clinics and doctors working in them were increasingly subjected to abuse and threats. Christian activists, such as Randall Terry, appeared to condone violence, but the Federal court insisted that these protests were justified as legitimate free speech. Then in March 1993 Michael Griffin, a committed member of the Assembly of God, shot dead the abortion doctor David Gunn. Several other shootings followed over the next eighteen months, until the Federal court reversed its decision. *Operation Rescue*, as this religiously inspired opposition to abortion was termed, was proscribed. In tracing this path of religious conviction against abortion leading eventually to such violence, *Wrath of Angels* provides a stark warning against easy assumptions about Christian compassion.

COMPASSION AND PVS PATIENTS

The ethically confusing situation of those carefully diagnosed as being in a so-called permanent, or at least persistent, vegetative state (PVS) provides a rather more sophisticated and lengthier

---

[35] James Risen and Judy L. Thomas, *Wrath of Angels: the American Abortion War* (New York: Basic Books, Perseus Book Group, 1999). See also Mark Juergensmeyer, *Terror in the Mind of God: the Global Rise of Violence* (Berkeley: University of California Press, 3rd edn, 2003), pp. 20f.

illustration of the significance of compassion in health care ethics. The issue of withdrawing nutrition and hydration from PVS patients has become deeply contentious, not just between Christians and secularists, but also among practising Christians, Jews and Muslims. Withholding and withdrawing nutrition and hydration has in the last few years been considered by both the Lambeth Conference of Bishops and by the Medical Ethics Committee of the British Medical Association. In both cases I was part of the discussion that preceded their respective reports,[36] although in neither case did I actually write the reports. Although their premises differed considerably, their main conclusions were very close. They offer a useful example of parallel Christian and secular discussions.

The Lambeth bishops defined their subject, agreed on a set of criteria and made recommendations based carefully upon them. It is, I believe, a model report which could be used widely in church and parish discussions, but which so far has been rather neglected.

The report identifies five 'bedrock principles upon which the discussion of euthanasia and related issues rest':[37]

- *Life is God-given and therefore has intrinsic sanctity, significance and worth.*
- *Human beings are in relationship with the created order and that relationship is characterised by such words as respect, enjoyment and responsibility.*
- *Human beings, while flawed by sin, nevertheless have the capacity to make free and responsible moral choices.*
- *Human meaning and purpose is found in our relationship with God, in the exercise of freedom, critical self-knowledge, and in our relationship with one another and the wider community.*
- *This life is not the sum total of human existence; we find our ultimate fulfilment in eternity with God through Christ.*

Having set out these principles, the bishops then reflect theologically and sensitively upon human pain and suffering and upon our responsibilities in Christ to other people. They are fully aware of

---

[36] See Robin Gill, *Moral Leadership in a Postmodern Age* (Edinburgh: T. & T. Clark, 1997), pp. 123–34.
[37] *The Official Report of the Lambeth Conference 1998* (Harrisburg, PA: Morehouse Publishing, 1999), pp. 101–2.

strong pressures in many countries to legalise *voluntary euthanasia* (i.e. 'where a competent, informed person asks another to end his or her life and is not coerced into doing so') and even *involuntary euthanasia* (e.g. 'where a terminally ill person, who does not have the capacity for informed choice, is killed').[38] Yet they believe that a combination of the first, second and fourth principles precludes either voluntary or involuntary euthanasia. They also worry about the consequential dangers of legalising such forms of euthanasia – especially the danger of abuse, the danger of diminution of respect for human life, and the danger of damaging the doctor/patient relationship. They take a firm stand against legalising euthanasia in these forms.

Yet they are also people with wide pastoral experience. Some of the bishops responsible for this report have direct experience of being hospital and hospice chaplains. As a result they are fully aware of the many ambiguous situations that modern medicine and technology can produce. For example, they believe that it is consonant with Christian faith for patients in some circumstances to refuse or terminate medical treatment. Christians do not, they argue on the basis of their fifth principle, need to cling to this life at all costs.

The bishops are also sympathetic to the House of Lords judgement of 3 February 1993 about the tragic Anthony Bland case. Bland was a victim of the Hillsborough football disaster. After being crushed by the crowd, he was in a PVS state for more than three years with no evident cortical activity (and thus without any cognition or sensation). His reflexes were still intact so he was able to breathe spontaneously, but he required intensive nursing – constantly being turned, receiving nutrition/hydration through a naso-gastric tube and being evacuated with enemas – in order to survive. After the legal judgement his naso-gastric tube was removed, he no longer received nutrition or hydration, and within two weeks he died from renal failure. The Lambeth bishops conclude that when such a person is safely diagnosed as PVS, then it can be right to withdraw life-prolonging medical treatment and medical intervention:

---

[38] The bishops derived their definitions from *Assisted Suicide and Euthanasia: the Washington Report* (Harrisburg, PA: Morehouse Publishing, 1997).

We have reached substantial agreement that the following measures are permissible and consonant with Christian faith:

- To withhold or withdraw excessive medical treatment or intervention (e.g. life support) may be appropriate where there is no reasonable prospect of recovery;
- When the primary intent is to relieve suffering and not to bring about death, to provide supportive care for the alleviation of intolerable pain and suffering (e.g. analgesics) may be appropriate even if the side effect of that care is to hasten the dying process;
- To refuse or terminate medical treatment (such as declining to undertake a course of chemotherapy for cancer) is a legitimate individual moral choice;
- When a person is in a permanent vegetative state, to sustain him or her with artificial nutrition and hydration may indeed be seen as constituting medical intervention.[39]

Representing a more pluralist constituency, the BMA Medical Ethics Committee report *Withholding and Withdrawing Life-Prolonging Medical Treatment* inevitably does not start from explicitly theological premises. Yet it does share the two main conclusions of the Lambeth bishops: namely, that public pressure to legalise voluntary euthanasia should be resisted, and that it can be right not to give life-prolonging treatment to patients when it simply becomes a burden to them. Essential to these conclusions is the BMA Medical Ethics Committee's initial understanding of the primary goal of medicine:

The primary goal of medical treatment is to benefit the patient by restoring or maintaining the patient's health as far as possible, maximising benefit and minimising harm. If treatment fails, or ceases, to give a net benefit to the patient (or if the patient has completely refused the treatment) that goal cannot be realised, and the justification for providing the treatment is removed. Unless some other justification can be demonstrated, treatment that does not provide net benefit to the patient may, ethically and legally, be withheld or withdrawn, and the goal of medicine should shift to the palliation of symptoms.[40]

Several conclusions follow naturally from this understanding. The BMA authors also believe that competent patients can properly refuse

---

[39] *The Official Report of the Lambeth Conference 1998*, p. 104.
[40] British Medical Association, *Withholding and Withdrawing Life-Prolonging Medical Treatment* (London: BMJ Books, 1999), para 1 (it was updated slightly in 2001 to take into account the Human Rights Act, although this paragraph remains unchanged).

treatment. In English law it has long been recognised that adults with the capacity to make decisions about their treatment do have the right to refuse life-prolonging, or even life-saving, treatment. So a competent and mature patient can properly refuse chemotherapy and opt for palliative care instead even if this effectively shortens her/his life. In such circumstances, doctors cannot legally act against such a patient's wishes. Again, doctors cannot give a life-saving blood transfusion to competent adult Jehovah's Witnesses who refuse (although they can sometimes give it against their wishes to their child).

However, like the bishops, the authors of the BMA report go further than this. They believe that medical treatment can properly be withdrawn from non-competent patients if it no longer offers them actual or potential benefit. This report argues that when people like Anthony Bland can no longer interact with others, are not aware of their existence, and can never again achieve purposeful action, then life-prolonging treatment does not provide them with any real benefit. It may, at that point, properly be withdrawn. In the case of babies born in similar conditions, life-prolonging treatment may properly be withheld altogether.

The BMA report is written with sensitivity. It recognises that families should be approached in a considerate and pastoral manner. Doctors should consult them, and other members of medical teams, carefully. Yet it is finally doctors, and not the courts (as at present in PVS cases), who ought, the report believes, to make medical decisions about withholding and withdrawing treatment.

However, there is an important difference between the two reports. The Lambeth bishops are more cautious about describing artificial forms of feeding as 'treatment'. Instead their report talks about 'medical intervention', since they are conscious that some people regard feeding, even in artificial forms, as a part of basic care and not as treatment. The BMA report, in contrast, argues that English law[41] already regards such feeding as treatment. For example, in the 1993 House of Lords judgement it was argued that the regime of naso-gastric feeding and evacuation using enemas that supported Anthony Bland does constitute 'a form of life support

---

[41] And similarly the American Supreme Court conclusion in the *Cruzan decision: Cruzan v Missouri Department of Health*, 110, Supreme Court 2481, 1990.

analogous to that provided by a ventilator which artificially breathes air in and out of the lungs of a patient incapable of breathing normally'. In the event, the bishops' distinction probably made little difference to their conclusions. On the basis of their pastoral experience, they accept that most of us simply do not want doctors to prolong our lives indefinitely, and to no purpose, with artificial forms of feeding. So, leaving it to others to decide whether artificial nutrition and hydration for PVS patients constitutes 'medical treatment' or 'medical intervention', the bishops too conclude that it can, in circumstances such as those facing Anthony Bland, properly be withdrawn.

A number of more purist religious groups remain strongly opposed to this conclusion (as was seen in the United States recently in the Terri Schiavo case), arguing that nutrition and hydration are a part of basic human care and should not be withdrawn from PVS patients at all. To withdraw, say, antibiotics from PVS patients may be allowable since this clearly constitutes 'treatment'. However, food and water should never be described as 'treatment' (or even 'intervention'), since if we withdraw them patients will certainly die. In contrast, if we withdraw 'treatment', patients, at most, will be allowed to die from their medical condition. Stated in this way it might seem that this purist group is more compassionate than either the BMA Medical Ethics Committee or the Lambeth bishops. They insist, after all, that it is our duty to offer patients basic care whatever their medical condition and however burdensome to society at large this might seem. True Christian, Jewish or Muslim care demands nothing less. This is what *agape* requires.

Perhaps the BMA report is too blunt in insisting that artificial forms of nutrition and hydration constitute 'medical treatment'. There may even be some sleight of hand at this point. Insisting that this is now established in English law, the report then assumes that it is thereby established in ethics as well. From that point onwards it is comparatively easy to show that there are many circumstances when it is morally right to withdraw treatment. Yet this is not a wise argument since the Anthony Bland case showed that law and ethics should not always be conflated so readily. Several of the English law lords showed that they were remarkably ill at ease in making their historic judgement precisely because they realised that the questions being raised went beyond their competence as lawyers and did involve serious moral issues. The academic lawyer Simon Lee[42] has exposed some of the weaknesses of their arguments at this very point, being particularly critical of the selective way Lord Hoffmann reached his ethical conclusions. Again, the Anthony Bland case revealed that the notions of withdrawing and withholding 'treatment' do not involve identical issues as is so often maintained. In this instance law and ethics pull in quite different directions. From a legal perspective it would undoubtedly have been easier if 'treatment' had been withheld from Anthony Bland in the first place rather than withdrawn three years later. Presumably this happened with other Hillsborough victims at the time, but this is seldom noticed. Yet from an ethical perspective initial 'treatment' was essential if it was to be properly established that Anthony Bland was in a persistent/permanent vegetative state. And some of us would maintain that, while it was ethically responsible to 'treat' in the first place, it was also ethically responsible (even if legally difficult) to withdraw this 'treatment' once a diagnosis of PVS had been safely established.

However, to depict the BMA report as lacking in compassion would thoroughly misrepresent it. The authors provide abundant evidence of their sensitivity and pastoral concern, as do the Lambeth bishops. Both doctors and bishops are aware that most people are anxious not to be sustained by means of medically delivered forms of nutrition and hydration indefinitely and to no purpose.

But is there really no purpose here? Religious purists typically use a second argument at this point, namely that withdrawing nutrition and hydration effectively involves involuntary euthanasia. For them there is little difference between ending the life of a PVS patient by means of an injection or by withdrawing nutrition and hydration. In both instances the patient dies and the doctor knows that this will happen. The only real difference is that withdrawing nutrition and hydration usually takes some two weeks to kill a patient, whereas an injection may be instantaneous. In contrast, withdrawing medical treatment, properly understood, simply allows the patient to die from her/his medical condition. There is, of course, an obvious weakness in the last part of this argument (to which I shall return

---

[42] Simon Lee, *Uneasy Ethics* (London: Pimlico, 2003).

in a moment), since withdrawing replacement forms of medical treatment from patients who cannot live without them (for example, withdrawing insulin from PVS diabetics) will just as effectively involve their death. And it could be argued that it was only artificial nutrition and hydration that prevented Anthony Bland from dying from his medical condition in the first place. These crucial points aside, there does seem to be a legitimate fear expressed by religious purists that the principle of not killing people is violated here.

Ironically, this conclusion is also reached by a number of non-religious ethicists championing voluntary euthanasia. They too con-clude that withdrawing nutrition and hydration from PVS patients violates the principle of not killing people. Yet, unlike the religious purists here, they welcome this violation. Len Doyal,[43] for example, argues that the withdrawal of life-sustaining treatment from perma-nently incompetent patients differs little morally from involuntary euthanasia (except that it prolongs possible suffering); it is already acceptable and allowed in Britain; so why is voluntary euthanasia not allowed as well? In logical terms, if we allow *a* then why do we not allow *b* (which is very similar), and if we then allow *b* why not *c* as well?

But another way of framing Doyal's argument is to say that the law must always draw a line at some point, and at the moment it is drawn between *a* and *b*. Of course the line could be moved (to after *b* or even after *c*), but that should, in my view,[44] only be done if we can be confident that the cost to the vulnerable and the common good will be less than if we left the line where it is at the moment.

The BMA report argues that there is a crucial difference between *a* and *b*:

Some people have argued that a doctor deciding to withdraw or withhold life-prolonging treatment (including, but not only, artificial nutrition and hydration) which will inevitably or very probably result in the patient's death *must* be doing so with the purpose or objective of ending that person's life. The BMA does not share this view. A doctor may withhold or withdraw life-prolonging treatment if the purpose of doing so is to withdraw treatment

---

[43] See the BMA public debate about euthanasia, 3 December 2003, on the web: http://www.bma.org.uk/ap.nsf/Content/MedicalEthicsTomorrowConfpapers
[44] See my response to Len Doyal in the BMA public debate.

which is not a benefit to the patient and is therefore not in the patient's best interest. In law, a doctor may foresee – be able to predict – that the patient will die if treatment is not provided, but this *cannot* be the sole reason for withholding it; the *overriding* purpose or objective is to ensure that treatment which is not in the best interests of the patient is avoided.[45]

The BMA report avoids a lengthy discussion of the troublesome doctrine of double effect,[46] yet it does once again conflate two languages, namely the ethical language of 'benefits' and the legal language of 'best interests'. Here too these languages may be more distinct than is allowed in the BMA report. The very notion of 'benefit' may expose ideological and metaphysical differences that, I suspect, the authors are anxious to avoid.

It is at this point that the Lambeth bishops may be better equipped to respond to those Christians, Muslims and Jews who object to their conclusions. From a theological perspective can it really be the case that sustaining PVS patients indefinitely constitutes a benefit either to them or to society at large? Once patients can no longer interact with others, are not aware of their existence, and can never again achieve purposeful action, then surely the BMA report is correct in claiming that life-prolonging treatment does not provide them with any real benefit. I believe that a theology of compassion suggests that it does not and that, once we regard people as children of God, then we have profound reasons why we should not burden such patients and their relatives beyond endurance even with our principled scruples. In terms of such theology, ethical principles are there to help and serve people, people are not there to serve principles. There are occasions when the vulnerable may need to be protected from an over-zealous application of principled scruples.

Of course this is a risky ethical stance to take. In the previous generation it was thoroughly misused by the Christian ethicist Joseph Fletcher, leading him to argue that all ethics is situational and that principles are at best relative guidelines.[47] But this is surely a *reductio*

---

[45] BMA, *Withholding*, para. 19.1.

[46] For a critique of double-effect in this context see Alastair Campbell's 'Response', in Robin Gill (ed.), *Euthanasia and the Churches* (London: Cassell, 1998), pp. 113–16: for a defence see Thomas Cavanaugh, 'Double Effect and the Ethical Significance of Distinct Volitional States', *Christian Bioethics*, 3:2 (1997), pp. 131–41.

[47] Joseph Fletcher, *Situation Ethics* (Philadelphia and London: Westminster and SCM Press, 1966).

ad absurdum. In contrast, a theology of compassion is concerned more with the vulnerable and with victims. It is closer to the risky form of ethics practised by Jesus in the Synoptic Gospels when he claimed that the Sabbath was made for people and not people for the Sabbath.

Once again Marcus Borg is helpful in understanding the tension within Christian ethics at this point: for him it involves a tension between the 'compassion code' and the 'holiness code'. For the pioneer Christian bioethicist William F. May it involves a tension between 'covenant' and 'contract' – a distinction which may be especially helpful in the contrasting roles of law and ethics in the withholding and withdrawing treatment debate. One Christian ethicist who did much to analyse this contrast was Joseph Allen, particularly in his book *Love and Conflict: a Covenantal Model of Christian Ethics.* For him a covenant model was significant for Christian ethics for three reasons. In the first place, it emphasises that human life is essentially social and that 'we are always dependent upon others and must entrust ourselves to them if we are to live at all and if we are to find what it is truly to live well'.[48] Secondly, 'a covenant model enables us to express the Christian awareness that each member of the covenant community has a value not reducible to his or her usefulness to the whole group'. And thirdly, a covenant model 'enables us to take seriously the *historical* fabric of the moral life, both of the individual and of the community, without losing our recognition of the moral unity of all people under God'.[49]

When Allen contrasted the model of covenant with that of contract in marriage its ethical importance can be seen most clearly. He argued as follows:

As a special covenant, marriage brings together a man and a woman in the most intensive relationship possible in human life. Their mutual concerns and obligations cover the whole range of life's interests, not merely a small or specific list of subjects, as might be the case in a business transaction. Once married, the two belong essentially together ... They will be able to sustain their marriage as a growing relationship only to the extent that they

---

[48] Joseph Allen, *Love and Conflict: a Covenantal Model of Christian Ethics* (Nashville: Abingdon Press, 1984), p. 46.
[49] Allen, *Love and Conflict,* p. 47.

commit themselves fully and steadfastly to each other and affirm each other as persons of worth, not only as individuals having convenient or useful or praiseworthy characteristics ... A covenant model of marriage is one that expresses the essential characteristics of covenant love in a way appropriate for this unique kind of human relationship. In contrast to a covenant model, much contemporary opinion views marriage as merely a limited-liability contract for the mutual advantage of each of the two spouses.[50]

Allen recognised that Christian marriage services typically contain a mixture of contractual and covenantal features, insisting that a valid marriage service requires the consent of both the man and the woman and that they have identifiable rights and corresponding obligations. Allen was not claiming that marriage as covenant eliminates the need for marriage as contract. Nevertheless he believed that marriage as covenant 'provides the theological framework within which the moral obligatoriness of the contract is to be understood, and not the reverse ... particular contractual matters within the marriage, however important, can be seen in their proper light – as means to the full affirmation of the other in marriage, and not as ways of pursuing private interests in competition with the marriage'.[51]

William F. May has argued for three decades that such a distinction between covenant and contract is important for a better understanding of the doctor–patient relationship. He has maintained that there are benefits in seeing this relationship in contractual terms 'in which two parties calculate their own best interests and agree upon some joint project in which they both derive roughly equivalent benefits for goods contributed by each'.[52] Such a model reduces doctor paternalism and stresses patient consent and doctor accountability. Nevertheless, for May 'it would be unfortunate if professional ethics were reduced to a commercial contract without significant remainder ... There is a donative element in the nourishing of covenant – whether it is the covenant of marriage, friendship, or

---

[50] Allen, *Love and Conflict*, p. 226.   [51] Allen, *Love and Conflict*, p. 227.

[52] William F. May, 'Code, Covenant, Contract or Philanthropy: a Basis for Professional Ethics', *Hastings Center Report* (December 1975), p. 33. See also his *The Physician's Covenant: Images of the Healer in Medical Ethics* (Philadelphia: Westminster Press, 1983). For a sympathetic critique see Gilbert Meilaender, 'On William May: Corrected Vision for Medical Ethics', in Allen Verhey and Stephen E. Lammers (eds.), *Theological Voices in Medical Ethics* (Grand Rapids, MI: William B. Eerdmans, 1993), pp. 114–19.

professional relationship . . . in which one must serve and draw upon the deepest reserves of another'.[53]

If contract is more to do with law and covenant with ethics, then perhaps the relationship between them in the withholding and withdrawing treatment debate becomes rather clearer. Both Allen and May have argued that covenant complements contract: contracts may be essential to ensure basic levels of justice but without covenantal behaviour they can become arid and lacking in compassion. So, whereas marriages lacking contracts can lead to injustice, marriages based solely upon contracts and without any covenantal love can result in joyless relationships. Writing in 1983 Allen feared that contractual understandings of marriage were too dominant. In the new millennium almost the reverse now seems to be the case. An increasing number of couples throughout the Western world are choosing to live together in a covenant but without a contract. This may allow romantic love to flourish, but ironically it may also increase injustice, especially for children.

The fine line required between rejecting voluntary or involuntary euthanasia and accepting, on occasions, withholding or withdrawing life-prolonging medical treatment and intervention, may require a similar delicate balance between contract and covenant. If contracts in this context are rightly concerned with principles, covenants are more concerned with relationships, especially with the vulnerable. In the Torah stories of covenant, God reaches out especially to people at moments of vulnerability – to Noah after the devastating flood, to Abraham and Sarah in apparently infertile old age and to Moses wandering in the wilderness. Unlike the mutuality of a good marriage, the terminally ill are more like the vulnerable recipients of God's covenants within the Torah. The terminally ill are in particular need both of protective principles and obligations and of genuine covenant/compassion. This, I believe, is the delicate balance required here.

Some theologians would go much further than me at this point. Both Paul Badham[54] and Hans Küng,[55] for example, have argued that voluntary euthanasia is compatible with Christian compassion.

[53] May, 'Code, Covenant, Contract', pp. 33–4.
[54] See Paul Badham, 'Should Christians Accept the Validity of Voluntary Euthanasia', in Gill, *Euthanasia and the Churches*, pp. 41–59.
[55] Hans Küng and Walter Jens, *A Dignified Dying* (London: SCM Press, 1995).

If someone who is terminally ill and in pain wishes to end her/his life, then Christian compassion may require that she/he should be helped to do so. Covenant theology, then, would be extended by them beyond withholding and withdrawing treatment or medical intervention. Elsewhere I have argued that, although there are important compassionate grounds for changing the law to allow for at least voluntary euthanasia (or 'physician-assisted suicide') for competent patients who are terminally ill and have intractable pain or distress,[56] such a change might have serious consequences for other vulnerable people as well as for the medical profession itself.[57] A fear of procedural deterioration – whereby exceptions for difficult cases become rights for all – has persuaded many of us that a well-meaning change in law might actually make the vulnerable more vulnerable. The situation in the Netherlands, in which doctors ending the lives of their patients still do not follow even the remarkably liberal Dutch procedures (for example, a significant number of euthanasia cases there are not reported, as required, and some do not even involve the terminally ill), does little to reduce this fear. Many politicians outside the Netherlands, Belgium and the State of Oregon still conclude that, if the vulnerable are to be properly protected, then the law does need to be clear and cautious. Legalising voluntary euthanasia, let alone legalising involuntary euthanasia, might, they believe, make serious abuse more likely than at present. Law and contract have a proper place here.

Nevertheless, there is abundant evidence from opinion polls that most people in Britain (and in other parts of the Western world), even many churchgoers, are unhappy with the present situation.[58] Not surprisingly most of us, given the choice, simply do not wish to have our lives sustained indefinitely when we can no longer interact with others, are not aware of our existence, and can never again achieve purposeful action. In such circumstances most of us probably agree that life-prolonging treatment or medical intervention would

---

[56] As Gilbert Meilaender concedes in his *Bioethics: a Primer for Christians* (Grand Rapids, MI: William B. Eerdmans, 1996), p. 65.

[57] See Robin Gill, 'Euthanasia – Response to Paul Badham', *Studies in Christian Ethics*, 11.1 (Edinburgh: T. & T. Clark, 1998), pp. 19–23.

[58] For these see Robin Gill, *Churchgoing and Christian Ethics* (Cambridge: Cambridge University Press, 1999), pp. 184f.

be a burden and not a benefit at all. However much we might hesitate about withdrawing nutrition and hydration from other people, few of us doubt that we would wish them to be withdrawn from ourselves in similar circumstances. The very thought of health care workers indefinitely prolonging us as empty shells, imprisoned in some scientifically created limbo, is abhorrent. Just as we regard enthusiasts of cryogenics as weird, most us are appalled by the thought that others might think it their principled duty to keep us 'alive' in the manner of Anthony Bland. When other people's principled scruples become a tyranny at our expense, then we are surely right to be worried.[59]

Inevitably the law becomes uneasy at this point. The diffidence of the English law lords in the Anthony Bland case is understandable. Nonetheless they were aware that it seemed devoid of compassion to sustain him in a persistent vegetative state indefinitely. However such an awareness is to be expressed in secular language, the notion of covenant is helpful at a theological level. It insists that for Jews, Christians and Muslims – sharing a fundamental conviction about God's overwhelming concern for all people – a concern for other people, and especially for the vulnerable, should be at the very heart of ethics.[60] More than that, the new covenant is not just some external law, but is actually written in people's hearts (Jeremiah 31.31–4).

A similar legal ambiguity is apparent even in palliative care. Of course good palliative care has helped doctors to be more discriminate and proportionate in their use, for example, of morphine. An earlier generation of doctors was less conscious of the difference between doses of morphine which were proportionate to treating pain and those which might directly shorten the life of the patient. The successful management of pain is a real achievement of palliative medicine. Notwithstanding this, there is still some ambiguity about when a dose of morphine, even if it is proportionate to pain, might contribute to shortening the life of a patient. The doctrine of double effect has frequently been invoked to justify this, but among a

---

[59] See Stephen Toulmin, 'The Tyranny of Principles: Regaining the Ethics of Discretion', *Hastings Center Report* (December 1981), and Kieran Cronin, *Rights and Christian Ethics* (Cambridge: Cambridge University Press, 1992), pp. 66f.

[60] See Garth Hallett, *Priorities and Christian Ethics* (Cambridge: Cambridge University Press, 1998).

number of ethicists and lawyers there are now considerable doubts about this doctrine. Properly understood, this doctrine insists that a foreseen but unintended secondary effect must not be wrong in itself – which is an obvious problem for those who believe that the medical shortening of life, whether intended or not, *is* wrong in itself. On strictly contractual grounds this aspect of palliative care may seem dubious. Yet on covenant grounds it does appear justifiable. Most people in severe pain do wish to receive powerful analgesics, even if they might shorten their lives. Genuine compassion, beyond contract, moves most doctors to respond. Indeed, a doctor who refused to give a patient morphine to ease severe pain, on the contractual ground that she/he risked prosecution, or even moral or theological approbation, for knowingly shortening life, would be applauded by few of us.

Good medicine does seem to require both contract and covenant. Perhaps the term 'covenant' itself is too theological for more general use within health care ethics. For Christians, Jews and Muslims it does carry the implication that human covenants are finally to be set in the context of God's generous and abundant covenant with us. The term 'compassion' may be able to unite people across religious and secular divides more readily. Oliver Davies has no problem in seeing a connection between compassion as a human virtue and compassion as a theological virtue, with the latter meaning much the same as the theological term 'covenant':

What we have argued . . . is that the presence of God with us is known to us through his acts of liberating compassion, and that this insight is given by God himself and is therefore of fundamental importance in our thinking about him. We have also suggested that the theological language of compassion serves in the main as a 'proper' or as a metaphorical name of God, rather than to remind us that we can only think about God in depth, and drawn near to him in understanding, where we re-enact within ourselves the conditions of his own being, which is to say dispossession of the self for the sake of the other. This is to begin to realize the symmetry that exists between his Trinitarian nature and the structure of our own consciousness, as the dialectical and mutually grounding relation of self and other.[61]

---

[61] Davies, *A Theology of Compassion*, p. 253.

Perhaps it really is time for health care ethics to be more explicit about the primacy of compassion. And perhaps it is also time for Christian bioethicists, especially when confronted with the vulnerable, to be more open to compassion trumping principled scruples.

CHAPTER 5

Care in health care ethics

The very title of this chapter signifies an important link between Christian and secular accounts of health care ethics. If 'care' is the second of the virtues present within the Synoptic healing stories, it is also a term with wide currency in secular medical contexts today – as in 'health care' itself, 'community care' and 'care assistants'. The health care professional is permitted and even expected to risk personal (but not intimate) contact with those who are ill or disabled and has a duty to do everything appropriate to cure them (if possible) or to reduce their pain or discomfort (if not) and, preferably, to eliminate the disease or condition itself. Care, properly understood, involves a range of core personal values, including competence, integrity, responsibility and confidentiality. Total patient care may also involve advocacy on behalf of the vulnerable and non-competent patient, as well as diligence to the common good and global justice.

Care, properly understood, is particularly demanding and highlights the gap between moral demands and human propensity to selfishness. In secular care one method adopted to ensure that adequate care is provided to patients is to produce written codes of professional practice and another is to have regular and systematic audits of actual practice. Using the recent writings of Onora O'Neill, it will be argued in the next chapter that such methods fall short of ensuring care, because care, properly understood, involves a personal relationship between a carer and a (conscious) patient. Written codifications and the written track records essential to audit, although important and certainly not to be denigrated, nevertheless tend to set out or test the minimum conditions for professional practice rather than the personal and compassionate care characterised in the Synoptic healing stories. Nonetheless there remain important features of secular medicine today that explicitly (and many more implicitly) contain care in the latter sense and that help to reduce the moral gap here.

The present chapter will argue that a specifically Christian account of 'care' adds an important, and sometimes neglected, critical tension between 'care' and 'compassion'. Because the latter is so often implicit rather than explicit in secular accounts of health care ethics, this critical tension can too easily be missed.

One of the few theologians to explore this critical tension in the context of health care ethics today is Margaret Farley. In her 2002 Madeleva Lecture in Spirituality[1] she sets out a concept of 'compassionate respect' that seeks to do justice to the demands of both compassion and care. She takes an extended example of responses to HIV/AIDS, to which this chapter will return shortly, arguing that 'compassion', although crucial for those living with HIV/AIDS, is nonetheless inadequate on its own to prevent the spread of this global pandemic. She could equally have taken as an example the increasing demand in many Western countries for the legalisation of voluntary euthanasia. Using the arguments of the previous chapter, it is not difficult to defend a compassionate case for legalised voluntary euthanasia for competent patients suffering from a terminal illness who are also experiencing intractable pain, suffering or distress. It might well be argued that vitalists defending an inviolate principle of the sanctity of life at the expense of such patients have simply failed to let compassion trump their principled scruples. A proper sense of compassion – understood as a response to the vulnerable and a determination to help them – does seem to support legalised voluntary euthanasia. Those campaigning for such a change in the law frequently, and quite properly, invoke compassion – for example, by encouraging courageous people like the British woman Dianne Pretty, shortly before her death from the effects of motor neuron disease, to make public appeals for their cause. Why should those with principled scruples be allowed to withhold compassionate deliverance from such vulnerable and terminally ill patients?

---

[1] Margaret A. Farley, *Compassionate Respect: A Feminist Approach to Medical Ethics and Other Questions* (New York and Mahwah, NJ: Paulist Press, 2002).

Once a wider notion of 'care' is taken into account, the answer to this question may not actually be straightforward. Now questions need to be asked about whether legalising voluntary euthanasia could be damaging to other vulnerable people. Will the frail elderly feel pressurised to have their lives ended? Will so-called procedural deterioration extend euthanasia to the partially competent or even to the non-competent? Will doctor–patient relationships be impaired, to the detriment of patients in general, by legalising voluntary euthanasia? Such questions suggest that there may be a critical tension between compassion for the individual patient and care of that patient in a context of other vulnerable people. If the former presents an overwhelming case for legalising voluntary euthanasia, the latter raises fears that legalising it for the few may make many other people more vulnerable. Or, as Margaret Farley argues, 'compassion requires at its core not only love but truth – not only the passion of compassion but the truth that compels respect'.[2]

In her account of a theologically derived 'compassionate respect', she sees important links with secular health care ethics:

a concern for compassion and its norms is parallel in many ways to debates in contemporary Western medical ethics about the relative adequacy of, on one hand, what is called an ethic of care and, on the other hand, what is identified as an ethic driven primarily by respect for individual patient autonomy.[3]

Drawing this parallel allows her to illustrate how 'autonomy' and 'care' – or 'compassion' and 'respect' – can be in critical, mutual tension with each other within a clinical context:

If, on the one hand, preoccupation with autonomy risks distorting our perception of the concrete needs of the patient for communication, companionship, assistance, and care – on the other hand, preoccupation with care, insofar as it fails to respect and even to foster autonomy, risks a return to the worst sorts of paternalism, mistaking harming for healing and the violation of bodily integrity for genuinely compassionate care . . . If care can be harmful or helpful, foolish or wise, mistaken or genuinely fitting, creative or destructive, what determines it to be one or the other? It must be that there are standards, criteria, measures for right caring, true caring, 'just' caring.[4]

---

[2] Farley, *Compassionate Respect*, p. 20.   [3] Farley, *Compassionate Respect*, pp. 20–2.
[4] Farley, *Compassionate Respect*, pp. 31–2.

Compassion needs to be expressed in care, and care, in turn, needs to be shaped by compassion. Compassion without care would soon be vacuous: care without compassion could soon become paternalistic and even harmful to the individual. If compassion 'draws us to persons, arrests our gaze and focuses it, so that we cannot pass by them in their need', then care holds us 'to the obligation that compassion awakens'.[5] Yet once care takes proper account of the wider context of those in need – that is of their needs and the needs of others – or, to express this differently, once care involves a notion of the common good, a creative tension can soon arise between care and compassion. Care understood as involving the common good might actually militate against compassion for particular individuals (notoriously so in democracies that pride themselves on being tolerant but then find it difficult to tolerate the intractably intolerant). Likewise compassion for particular individuals may preclude the possibility of ever reaching a resolution of some common good issues (notoriously those concerned with environmental sustainability).

The Synoptic healing stories illustrate such tension at several points. There is sometimes a tension between compassion and anger. There can be a tension between individual touching and ritual purity – a tension between the individual and the communal and between respecting purity laws and infringing them. And there can be a tension between compassionate care for a vulnerable individual and care for the wider community. Creative tension runs through these healing stories.

Mark's story of the cleansing of the leper can again be taken to illustrate some of these tensions:

1.40 A leper came to him begging him, and kneeling he said to him, 'If you choose, you can make me clean.' 41 Moved with pity, Jesus stretched out his hand and touched him, and said to him, 'I do choose. Be made clean!' 42 Immediately the leprosy left him, and he was made clean. 43 After sternly warning him, he sent him away at once, 44 saying to him, 'See that you say nothing to anyone, but go, show yourself to the priest, and offer for cleansing what Moses commanded, as a testimony to them.'

As argued earlier, compassion is clearly involved in this story. If the NRSV is followed, it is explicitly present in the first words of verse 41

---

[5] Farley, *Compassionate Respect*, p. 80.

(using the verb *splankgnizesthai*, itself derived from the Greek word for 'bowels', i.e. the traditional seat of emotion). If the variant reading of 'anger' rather than 'pity' is followed here, it is still present implicitly in Jesus' prompt response to the leper's begging plea. And if 'anger' is not allowed here, it is explicit in the first words of verse 43. Jesus evidently cares passionately about this leper and, of course, chooses to touch him despite his evident impurity. This, in turn, is followed by a concern to abide by the societal concerns for ritual cleansing (as in Luke 17.18). In short, the story moves from an individual compassion directed at this particular leper, through caring concern, contact and cleansing, to a socially proscribed ritual.

James Dunn warns against making too easy a paradox here: namely, that Jesus first defies purity laws by touching the leper and then keeps them by referring the cleansed leper to the priest to make an offering. Instead Dunn stresses that it was not wrong or sinful for a Jew to contract impurity:

On the contrary, the son of a parent who died was duty bound to contract impurity in attending to his father's burial; the impurification caused by discharges from the sexual organs did not make the menstruating woman a sinner or require abstinence from sexual intercourse. So we cannot say that Jesus touched the leper (1.41) in defiance of the purity code. And the probable testimony of 1.44 is that Jesus instructed the leper to follow the required procedure for a person with a contagious skin disease to be readmitted to society. In which case Jesus acted in accord with the purity laws.[6]

Nonetheless, Dunn does finally detect a crucial ambivalence in the Synoptic Jesus' response to purity. For him, 'the point is rather that Jesus seems to disregard the impurity consequences in such cases, so that it may be fairly concluded that Jesus was indifferent to such purity issues'.[7] And again, 'the fact that he sat loose to the purity *halakhoth* regarding clean and unclean table-fellowship suggests equally, if not more strongly, that he did not regard such concerns as central to his understanding of what constituted the Israel of God and what should regulate Jews' social praxis of their religion'.[8]

---

[6] James D. G. Dunn, 'Jesus and Purity: an Ongoing Debate', *New Testament Studies*, 48 (2002), p. 461.
[7] Dunn, 'Jesus and Purity', p. 461.   [8] Dunn, 'Jesus and Purity', p. 467.

If Dunn is right about all of this, it does seem to be compatible with an approach in Christian ethics that is prepared, when required by compassion, to trump principled scruples, but that, when this is not required, does still observe these scruples in the interests of a wider context of care. Clearly there is an uneasy tension here – there was after all no guarantee that Jewish purity laws, which might on occasions have been properly disregarded, might, on other occasions and in a wider setting, have been socially beneficial (the early Christians, after all, were soon to conclude that the latter was not the case). Yet it is a tension that, in other forms, can still characterise modern clinical situations. Just think, for example, of the uneasy tolerance of infant male circumcision in modern medicine. It is often argued that it is difficult to justify male circumcision, for all but a few infants, using the evidential criteria of modern physical medicine,[9] yet it is still tolerated (albeit with considerable dissent) on social, communal or religious/traditional grounds. In most other circumstances, an irreversible medical intervention lacking both patient consent and clear medical benefit, would not be tolerated at all. After all, the traditional African practice of female circumcision (notwithstanding its maleficence compared with male circumcision) is now proscribed on compassionate grounds in much modern medicine. Yet, for the moment and with many qualms, infant male circumcision remains a legal, clinical option even in the West.

Luke's parable of the good or compassionate Samaritan (10.25–37) offers a particularly detailed illustration of the interplay of compassion and care. It is the first of his unique and lengthy narrative parables, it is written in an unusually literary style, uncharacteristically for a parable it relates directly to healing, and it has been (and remains) surprisingly influential even within secular health care ethics.

Compassion is the prime mover of this parable. It is of course the heterodox Samaritan, and not the priest or the Levite, who, rather than passing by on the other side, 'when he saw him … was moved with pity' (10.33). For Evans, '*Samaritan* is probably chosen as the traditional enemy, one who as a schismatic is excluded from the covenant fellowship of neighbours (i.e. Israelites), but who, in

---

[9] Although see R. V. Short, 'Male Circumcision: a Scientific Perspective: the Health Benefits of Male Circumcision are Wide Ranging', *Journal of Medical Ethics*, 30:3 (2004), p. 241.

contrast to the embodiments and representatives of the covenant people, carries out the requirements of the covenant'.[10] The verb *splankgnizesthai* is again explicitly used here ('moved with pity'). To reinforce this the lawyer at whom the parable is directed identifies the Samaritan as 'the one who showed him mercy [*eleos*]' (10.37) and the parable itself is prefaced by the command to love 'your neighbour as yourself' (10.27). The whole fits exactly the understanding of compassion as a response to the vulnerable and a determination to help them. The man has been stripped, beaten and left half-dead: it is the Samaritan who responds to this vulnerable stranger and he alone who shows a determination to help him. It is this core element of the parable that still survives in secular health care ethics. The off-duty doctor who responds to a call for medical help on a flight or at the roadside is still identified with the good Samaritan. Ironically today it is less a fear of possible pollution from a half-dead stranger (as Jeremias suggested)[11] that is likely to deter a doctor today from acting the good Samaritan than a fear of subsequent litigation for having acted negligently.

Having shown compassion, the Samaritan immediately responds with compassionate care. There is none of the anger here that is so characteristic of Synoptic healing stories, but there is touching and considerable after-care. In turn the Samaritan:

- Went to him
- Bandaged his wounds
- Poured oil and wine on them
- Put him on his own animal
- Brought him to an inn
- Took care of him
- Gave two denarii to the innkeeper
- Said 'Take care of him'
- And said 'I will repay you whatever more you spend'

Of course today oil and wine would not be regarded as appropriate medication for wounds, medical or paramedical expertise would be

---

[10] C. F. Evans, *Saint Luke* (London and Philadelphia: SCM Press and Trinity Press, 1990), p. 469.
[11] J. Jeremias, *The Parables of Jesus* (London: SCM Press, 1963). But see Evans, *Luke*, p. 468 for dissent.

required before moving a patient suffering from trauma, an ambulance would definitely be preferred to animal transport, the patient would be brought not to an inn but to an Accident and Emergency Unit and the latter might or might not require immediate payment (different perhaps in the US to the UK)! Nonetheless, the overall structure of care is remarkably similar. In the holistic terms of modern Systems Pastoral Care,[12] it is the person as a social being, and not simply the physical wounds, who needs to be cared for and tended.

The critical tension in this parable appears early and is implicitly caused by the differing responses of the priest, the Levite and the Samaritan. It is not difficult to imagine how, in a context of long-standing anti-clericalism, especially in Catholic Europe, this parable might be interpreted. Within this context the image of the priest who lacks all compassion may resonate strongly: it is the ordinary person outside the 'established church' who shows genuine compassionate care. As the popular saying goes 'You don't have to go to church to be a good Christian' or, more appropriately, 'You don't have to be religious to be good' or perhaps, especially after 9/11, 'Religion causes more harm than good.'

In Luke's parable of the prodigal son (15.11–32) critical tension is set at the very juncture between 'compassion' and 'care' and is quite explicit. It is possible to read this parable, too, as being relevant to healing. Evans, for example, concludes:

The point of the parable would ... seem to be, not the penitence and conversion of the sinner as such (generally in the gospels they are presumed rather than described), but the miraculous fact that these occur, and that they are equivalent to life from the dead. The only defect of the dutiful son, who is the permanent sharer of the father's company and possessions, is to fail to appreciate the miracle, and the unfairness which, by ordinary standards, it entails.[13]

The central tension in this parable is indeed created by the relationship of the two sons to the father and his relationship to them. It is the father who 'was filled with compassion' for the younger son

---

[12] See E. Mansell Pattison, 'Systems Pastoral Care', *The Journal of Pastoral Care*, 26:1 (1972), pp. 3–14.
[13] Evans, *Luke*, p. 591.

(15.20: once again the verb *splankgnizesthai*) and it is the elder son who 'became angry and refused to go in' (15.28). In between the compassion and the anger are a series of acts of compassionate care by the father:

- He ran and put his arms around him
- He kissed him
- He ordered the best robe to be put on him
- A ring to be put on his finger
- Sandals on his feet
- The fatted calf to be killed
- And for people to eat and celebrate

Famously these acts of compassionate care are simply provocative to the dutiful son. His perennial response is:

Listen! For all these years I have been working like a slave for you, and I have never disobeyed your command: yet you have never given me even a young goat so that I might celebrate with my friends. But when this son of yours came back, who has devoured your property with prostitutes, you killed the fatted calf for him! [15.29–30]

Compassionate care for one son causes passionate resentment in the other.

By adding a few embellishments to the parable of the good Samaritan it is possible to manufacture similar tensions there between the different claims of compassion and care. Suppose, for example, that the victim of the violence was actually a violent and ruthless exploiter of the poor in the region. Far from being an innocent victim of brutal thieves, he was in reality a merciless brigand who had at last got his comeuppance from the poor whom he had exploited. The Samaritan still acts – as doctors today should do – because the brigand, even one who showed no compassion to others, is in serious need of care and may die without it. Yet by acting in this way the Samaritan offends the local people who believe that the brigand has at last got his just deserts. Or suppose the parable, in line with modern Systems Pastoral Care, is extended to take account of subsequent political action. So now the Samaritan, once assured that the victim is being cared for at the inn, seeks to make the road from Jerusalem and Jericho safe from robbers. At once he faces a serious and contentious choice of campaigning either for stronger deterrents against, or for economic relief for, would-be robbers. He might even adopt a more traditional Marxist approach and question the assumptions about private property that underpin notions of 'theft', seeking to persuade local sceptics that they should not be possessive about 'their' property and that thieves are really not 'thieves' at all.

Of course it is anachronistic to embellish the details of Synoptic parables in this way. These fanciful conjectures simply make the point that 'compassion' and 'care', although mutually dependent in an adequate understanding of health care ethics, can nonetheless be in critical tension with each other.

David Hollenbach's *The Common Good and Christian Ethics* helps to clarify this tension further. Hollenbach has been an influence upon the widely discussed social pronouncements of the American Catholic bishops in recent years. In his important contribution to New Studies in Christian Ethics, he seeks to defend the Catholic notion of 'the common good', starting with Aristotle:

> One of Aristotle's most significant conclusions was that a good life is oriented to goods shared with others – the common good of the larger society of which one is a part. The good life of a single person and the quality of the common life persons share with one another in society are linked. Thus the good of the individual and the common good are inseparable. In fact, the common good of the community should have primacy in setting direction for the lives of individuals, for it is a higher good than the particular goods of private persons.[14]

Yet he is well aware of the difficulties that a notion of the common good faces in modern pluralistic, democratic societies. There is the long-standing fear engendered by the religious wars of the sixteenth and seventeenth centuries that still find parallels in tensions between Christians and Muslims in various parts of the world and specifically between Hindus and Muslims in India, between Catholics and Protestants in Northern Ireland and between Jews and Muslims in Israel. All too often in the past and in the present the 'common' good has been imposed by one religious group upon another through coercion rather than mutually agreed through dialogue. There is

---

[14] David Hollenbach, *The Common Good and Christian Ethics* (Cambridge: Cambridge University Press, 2002), p. 3.

also the self-evident cultural pluralism of modern democratic societies (especially, as was seen earlier, among health care professionals
drawn as they are now in the West from all parts of the world), with
sharp differences within and between religious and secular groups.

In other words, Hollenbach is well aware of the moral gaps
identified in the first chapter, especially the gap between theoretical
and actual moral communities and the gap between personal resonance and a shared understanding of cosmic order. In a traditional
society there may well be a shared sense of cosmic order and an
identifiable moral community that together make possible a viable
sense of common good. However, in a modern society, still shaped by
a fear of past religious wars, but now also experiencing considerable
cultural pluralism as a result of increasing globalisation, such a sense
is considerably more problematic.

Given this modern social milieu, Hollenbach explores the idea that
it is individualistic values such as tolerance that now constitute the
point of commonality in the Western world:

There are many indications in the United States today that tolerance of
diversity occupies the place held by the common good in the thought of
Aristotle, Thomas Aquinas and Ignatius Loyola. Tolerance of difference, not
the common good, has become the highest social aspiration in American
culture. And the range of matters to which tolerance is extended has been
broadening.[15]

Hollenbach argues that this raises fundamental questions:

Will a culture in which tolerance is the prime virtue generate a society good
enough to sustain its citizens' loyalty over the long haul? Does avoiding
judgments lead to an attenuated vision of what is possible by telling us never
to say anything in public that others do not already agree with? If tolerance
becomes a card that trumps all other strong proposals on how we should live
together, will it stifle the imagination needed to address pressing public
problems?[16]

His book argues at length that individualistic values such as
tolerance on their own are simply not adequate to resolve all of the
social dilemmas of modern democratic societies. He cites at length
two areas that particularly demonstrate this inadequacy. The first

---

[15] Hollenbach, *Common Good*, p. 24.　　[16] Hollenbach, *Common Good*, p. 31.

concerns the enduring poverty and inequality that characterise size-able minorities especially within American cities. He argues that it is not racial prejudice as such that is the primary causal factor of inner-city poverty and thus it is not racial tolerance that is its solution:

> Deprivation caused by economic inequality and class divisions will not be addressed directly or adequately by increasing the level of racial tolerance in society. Acceptance of racial differences within a commitment to our common humanity must surely be pursued in its own right. Nothing said here should be taken to suggest otherwise. But the virtue of tolerance, by itself, is not now a sufficient moral resource for addressing the problems of the poor in America's core cities. Toleration alone will not overcome class divisions and the despair they engender among the poor. Addressing these problems in a serious way will require reflection on the barriers that isolate the inner-city poor from both the white and the black middle classes in the suburbs. It will also mean concerted efforts to overcome these class barriers. Tolerance means *acceptance* of difference, perhaps even a kind of *acquiescence* in such differences.[17]

So, tolerance *is* important for Hollenbach. But it is not sufficient. And, taken in isolation, it may even promote acquiescence and impede a solution to this social issue.

The second area relates to global issues[18] that affect people across class and ethnic groups both nationally and internationally:

> Trade, finance, mass communications, the interaction of cultures, protection of the environment, the AIDS crisis, and the reality of poverty are all matters that have increasingly global dimensions. Today, economic, cultural, and political affairs occur within networks of human interaction that stretch across national borders. An ethos whose primary values are independence and autonomy is not adequate to address this new interdependence. Such an ethos systematically avoids attending to the impact of human interconnections on the quality of life by focusing on the freedom and choices of individuals one at a time. When the possibility of attaining good lives and freedom itself are becoming more dependent on new interconnections, however, much more attention must be given to the way the well-being of individuals is shaped by institutional connections with others.

---

[17] Hollenbach, *Common Good*, p. 40.
[18] See also William Schweiker, *Theological Ethics and Global Dynamics: In the Time of Many Worlds* (New York and London: Blackwell, 2004).

Globalization is thus challenging the received tradition of public values that has prevailed in the West for the past several centuries.[19]

This raises very serious problems for privileged individuals within the West. A concern for the wider consequences of globalisation may actually curtail their individual freedoms. For example, a concern about environmental destruction may curtail the consumption of individuals, so that, in the interests of the 'common good' (but not in the interests of their own immediate good), they use less fossil fuels to travel or to heat/cool their houses. In both areas Hollenbach argues that the notion of the common good adds dimensions of mutual respect and interrelatedness that are not present in such individual-istic values as tolerance or autonomy.

Hollenbach argues that churches have an important role to play in contributing to the common good even within pluralistic societies and that they have indeed made such a contribution in a number of modern societies. He believes that there is evidence 'that indicates that active participation by citizens in public life is seriously threat-ened today and that religious communities possess distinctive capa-cities to enhance such citizenship'.[20] Emphatically he does not believe that churches and their theologians should address their concerns only to fellow Christians, maintaining that there are good theological reasons for believing that public activity is a proper function of churches. In arguing for this position he is well aware that he is seeking to counter currently popular exclusive theologians, as well as secular philosophers, who consider theology to be irrelevant to the public forum today (in my terms he is a theological realist rather than a theological purist):

Christians, of course, should go forward in partnership and dialogue with those holding other religious convictions and with non-believers as well. This work, though, calls for Christians to speak forth what they believe and hope about where the full common good lies. If they do so with the right combination of courage and humility, this will help bring the full common good closer for all.[21]

---

[19] Hollenbach, *Common Good*, pp. 42–3.   [20] Hollenbach, *Common Good*, p. 88.
[21] Hollenbach, *Common Good*, p. 243.

CARE AND THE CHALLENGE OF HIV/AIDS

The complex relationship between compassion and care can be illustrated at greater length by considering ethical responses both to the plight of the millions of people now living with HIV/AIDS and to the daunting epidemiological problem of how to contain and limit the global spread of this deadly virus. It does not take long to discover that there is a serious tension between these two sets of ethical responses. If the first requires compassion and care for those living with HIV/AIDS, the second may require passionate, caring political/social action that is sometimes at odds with individual compassion and care.

There are obvious affinities between leprosy in biblical times (whether or not it actually was leprosy in a modern sense) and HIV/AIDS in sub-Saharan Africa today. In both contexts it was incurable and even palliative treatment was unavailable for most of its victims. Those living with leprosy or HIV/AIDS were both objects of considerable stigma and social exclusion. There was much fear about physical contact with both. Both involved notions of impurity as well as untouchability. There were deep suspicions that both were the products of sinful behaviour. Both were seen by some as instruments of God's/fate's judgement. And both required repentance from the one suffering rather than compassion from other people.

Drawing on his long experience in south India, the Methodist theologian Eric Lott uses the story of the leper in the opening chapter of Mark to reflect powerfully upon the life of lepers and Dalits today. Leprosy is endemic in a part of India where he lived for many years, 'so the sight of men and women alarmingly disfigured by this disease, with face, fingers, feet ravaged almost beyond recognition as parts of a human body, sometimes with no fingers at all – lost through repeated injuries and infection from lack of feeling – such a sight was almost a daily occurrence'.[22] World-wide some 15 million people still live with leprosy. For Lott, the plea from the leper in Mark reminds him:

Leprosy was, and still is often, so dreaded, that the leper was regarded as already as good as dead. Leprosy is so abhorrent to people that its very

---

[22] Eric Lott, *Healing Wings: Acts of Jesus for Human Wholeness* (Bangalore, India: Asian Trading Corporation, 1998), p. 39.

existence is ignored, the presence of lepers, singly or in groups, is just not recognised. Many times I have watched people walking along a city street apparently just not seeing the presence of a leper begging straight in front of them. No doubt this can be a protective measure: 'Show the slightest interest and you'll be pestered to death. And in any case we must discourage all begging, must we not?' But it runs deeper than that. The very term 'leper' has come to mean one who is shunned, ostracised because he is polluting, outcast because he is dangerously cursed.[23]

In India, leprosy is still commonly (and mistakenly) believed to be both virulently infectious and incurable. And, even worse, is the fear that 'this disease is a curse from God, or is the result of one's *karma*, the outworking of some heinous deed done in a past life ... all you can do is submit to this self-created fate'.[24]

Lott notes the anger of Jesus in Mark's story and compares it with the occasions 'when the disciples tried to stop little children from being brought for a blessing; when over-pious Pharisees condemned ordinary people as being outside the good purpose of God; when ritualist Priests prevented non-Jews from praying at the Temple, by making the Court set aside for them a market-place'.[25] And he links this to the situation of the Dalits (the so-called 'untouchables') in India today. Especially, he notes the touching, arguing that 'Jesus, in this act of stretching out his hand to touch a polluted leper, shouts loud and clear that we are *wrong*; this way of thinking is against the Spirit of God; we contradict the ways of God's new world by this fear that any of God's children are polluting.'[26]

In all of this Lott might also have been referring to the emaciated figures of those living with the later stages of AIDS in sub-Saharan Africa today. Those of us who have been to sub-Saharan Africa recently (with some 28 million living with HIV/AIDS), as well as to southern India, will recognise the poignant similarities at once. And tragically HIV/AIDS is now spreading in India as well.

A focus upon those living with leprosy is a distinctive feature of the Synoptic Gospels and of Luke in particular. There is no mention of this disease elsewhere in the New Testament. Altogether there are six discrete references to it in the Synoptic Gospels. One of these is

---

[23] Lott, *Healing Wings*, pp. 40–1.   [24] Lott, *Healing Wings*, p. 41.
[25] Lott, *Healing Wings*, p. 43.   [26] Lott, *Healing Wings*, p. 46.

curious and difficult to interpret, namely the mention of Jesus being 'in the house of Simon the leper' when a woman anoints him with costly ointment (Mark 14.3 and Matt. 26.6). Vincent Taylor suggested prosaically that this house 'must have been known to the circle from which the story comes'[27] ... a bit like referring to 'the Jew's House' in Lincoln today. Or perhaps this is yet another occasion when Jesus is depicted as associating with the 'impure'. Whatever the explanation, a common feature of the other five references is that each refers explicitly to 'cleansing' and, by doing so, identifies leprosy with 'impurity'. All three Synoptic Gospels have the story of the cleansing of the leper (Mark 1.40–5 / Matt. 8.1–4 / Luke 5.12–16). However, Luke embellishes the story by depicting him as 'a man covered with leprosy' (5.12). In Matthew the twelve disciples are charged to 'cure the sick, raise the dead, cleanse the lepers, cast out demons' (10.8). In both Matthew and Luke, John the Baptist's disciples are told to report back that 'the blind receive their sight, the lame walk, the lepers are cleansed, the deaf hear, the dead are raised, (and) the poor have good news brought to them' (Matt. 11.5 and Luke 7.22). And Luke alone first makes an allusion to the cleansing of Naaman the leper (4.27) and then recounts the story of the cleansing of the ten lepers (17.11–19).

This strong association of leprosy with cleansing/impurity is also part of a wider picture in the Synoptic Gospels. Just to take Mark alone, there are additional healing stories about a man in the synagogue with an 'unclean spirit' (1.23), about a crowd with 'unclean spirits' (3.11), the Gerasene demoniac with an 'unclean spirit' (5.2), the Syro-Phoenician woman's daughter with an 'unclean spirit' (7.25) and an epileptic boy with an 'unclean spirit' (9.25). In two of these stories Jesus is also depicted as deliberately touching those regarded as 'unclean'.

Given this distinctive focus, it may not be too surprising that health care in modern India has been disproportionately delivered through Christian agencies. Although (outside Kerala, Goa and Assam) Christians remain a very small proportion of the Indian population, they form a sizeable group particularly among nurses. It is possible that this Synoptic focus upon those living with leprosy

[27] Vincent Taylor, *The Gospel According to St Mark* (London: Macmillan, 1959), p. 530.

and other 'unclean' diseases and disabilities, together with accounts of Jesus deliberately disregarding their impurity consequences, has had an abiding influence upon Indian Christians. Unlike many of their Hindu contemporaries, they belong to a culture that has long questioned deep-set notions of 'purity' and 'impurity' in a context of compassionate care. So among Christian families in India nursing tends to be encouraged, just as it is in the Western world. It is regarded, not so much as an occupation tainted by impurity (involving, as it necessarily does, contact with intimate bodily parts and fluids), but as a respectable, caring profession. And this is the case not just among the Dalit community – who traditionally undertook tainted occupations and who are now disproportionately Christian – but more generally among Indian Christian families. The social perception of nursing has been reconfigured beyond notions of 'purity' and 'impurity' that are still dominant in wider Indian culture. A rather striking example of Christian socialisation.

A similar process seems increasingly to have influenced attitudes towards those living with HIV/AIDS. Two decades ago leaders in some churches identified the virus as God's punishment of the gay community (when it was thought to be a disease only affecting that community) and then of general sexual promiscuity. A gradual realisation that the virus also affected haemophiliacs who had been given infected blood, their spouses, and even their babies, together with a more compassionate approach to others living with HIV/AIDS often in conditions of extreme poverty, began to marginalise this initial identification. Perhaps also more careful reflection upon such texts as John 9.2–3 ('His disciples asked him. "Rabbi, who sinned, this man or his parents, that he was born blind?" Jesus answered, "Neither this man nor his parents sinned"'), together with the force of the Synoptic healing stories, encouraged this change.

Margaret Farley writes of a growing inter-religious agreement about the need for a compassionate approach to those living with HIV/AIDS. At a major international (and predominantly African) conference of religious leaders on World AIDS Day in December 2000 she found that 'the words of compassion were inspiring and uncontroversial':[28]

---

[28] Farley, *Compassionate Respect*, p. 9.

Imams, rabbis, patriarchs, archbishops, sheikhs, and many others came to the conference together from the nations of the South to consider together what an effective religious response could be. One after another they spoke of how they had become aware of the problem of HIV/AIDS in their own geographical situations. One after another they articulated in terms of their own contexts the need for compassion. The shared experience of rising compassion was almost palpable. It included reports of compassionate responses on the part of faith communities to those vulnerable to and suffering from AIDS. Religious groups, it was noted, are caring for the dying and for the living, and they have begun the work of prevention and even advocacy for the needs of their people.[29]

Lisa Cahill, like Farley a feminist Roman Catholic theologian, outlines in some detail ways that churches have recently played a significant part in advocacy networks concerned with HIV/AIDS. As noted in chapter 1, she argues that advocacy for social justice is one of the major (and sometimes unnoticed) ways that churches have been socially influential in the modern world. More than that, for her the distinctive contribution of religion in health care ethics *should* be to emphasise social justice in access to medical benefits. She specifically claims that 'a striking example from the health care realm is a series of events that in about a two-year period loosened the grip of major pharmaceutical companies on patented AIDS drugs, making them available cheaply or for free in countries with high rates both of poverty and of AIDS deaths'.[30] In South Africa, in particular, 'religious voices, local activism, NGOs, the U.N., market competition from generic drug manufacturers, and market pressure from consumers and stockholders all played some part, resulting in a modification of World Trade Organization policy on intellectual property, over which the power of big business had seemed unassailable at the start'.[31] In a recent *Hastings Center Report* she sets out in detail the complex process of lobbying, political activism and litigation in South Africa that made this possible. At the time of the crucial trial at the Pretoria High Court in 2001, when the Pharmaceutical Manufacturers Association of South Africa attempted unsuccessfully

[29] Farley, *Compassionate Respect*, p. 7.
[30] Lisa Sowle Cahill, 'Bioethics, Theology, and Social Change', *Journal of Religious Ethics*, 31:3 (2003), p. 385.
[31] Cahill, 'Bioethics, Theology, and Social Change', p. 386.

to challenge the use of cheap generic drugs to combat AIDS, 'pro-testers were led in prayer by the Roman Catholic archbishop and the Anglican bishop, who said, "we can't on the one hand look at the sanctity of human life and on the other hand have these drugs that are not affordable to the people"'.[32] This example convinces Cahill that 'the lesson for theological bioethics is that social change is possible even when the entrenched systems of control over goods are infected with structural sin'.[33]

Church-related advocacy and activism on HIV/AIDS are now taking a variety of forms. In San Francisco, which witnessed some of the earliest known deaths from AIDS, the Episcopalian Grace Cathedral has had an Interfaith AIDS Memorial Chapel since 1995. The triptych in this chapel, *The Life of Christ*, was completed five years earlier by the gay artist Keith Haring two weeks before he died of AIDS. In a glass case there is a handmade Book of Remembrance with the names of people who have died from AIDS inscribed within it. An AIDS Memorial Quilt, representing tens of thousands of people around the country, is also rotated and expanded by volun-teers at regular intervals. The chapel has its aim to be 'a space for remembrance and celebration', identifying the cathedral itself with AIDS advocacy.

The World Council of Churches has also long been involved in AIDS advocacy. At a time when some church leaders were indeed still identifying the virus as God's punishment, the WCC executive committee in 1987 instead affirmed 'that God deals with us in love and mercy and that we are freed from simplistic moralizing about those who are attacked by the virus'.[34] In 1994 the WCC's central committee, meeting in Johannesburg, mandated the formation of a consultative group to conduct a study on HIV/AIDS. The study document that resulted from this, *Facing AIDS: the Challenge, the Churches' Response*, was first published in 1997 and has been reprinted many times since. It argued that 'churches have a distinctive and crucial role to play in facing the challenges raised by HIV/AIDS', but

---

[32] Lisa Sowle Cahill, 'Biotech Justice: Catching up with the Real World Order', *Hastings Center Report*, 33:5 (2003), p. 40.

[33] Cahill, 'Bioethics, Theology, and Social Change', p. 386.

[34] Quoted in *Facing AIDS: The Challenge, the Churches' Response* (Geneva: World Council of Churches Publications, 1997), pp. 102–3.

Before answering these two questions, a brief thought experiment might help. At the time of his death in 1989 it was claimed that the French novelist Georges Simenon had slept with some 10,000 women during his life-time. There is obviously no way to verify this, but suppose for the moment that it is accurate and then suppose that half of these women were prostitutes (he admitted to using prostitutes). Suppose again that the 5,000 prostitutes had a modest 1,000 clients each per year and worked on average for ten years each. In theory, at least, they had a combined score of 50,000,000 sexual contacts (rather more than the total male population of France). Suppose, in contrast, the 5,000 non-prostitutes who slept with Simenon only slept with a further two men. In theory they had a combined score of 10,000, but in reality they were directly connected through Simenon (assuming that he eschewed condoms) with the enormous score of the prostitutes. If Simenon himself had been infected with the HIV virus, then all 50,010,000 would theoretically have been at risk (although of course it cannot be assumed that in reality these were all separate individuals). And even if all 5,000 non-prostitute women had remained faithful to a single partner after their encounter with Simenon, the score of theoretical sexual contacts would still be 50,005,000. Even if this total is hopelessly exaggerated and needs to be reduced ten-fold, it still amounts to over five million interlinked sexual contacts. In epidemiological terms (even before the emergence of HIV/AIDS) such a conjunction of bodily fluids presents a very serious risk of infection. From such a thought experiment, focused upon the claims about a single individual, it is easy to see how hundreds of truck drivers using prostitutes along the trade roads from Angola and Mozambique have had such a devastating role in spreading the HIV virus through southern Africa.

To return to the two questions relating to stigmatisation and notifiability, the answer is surely that a positive response would conflict seriously with the compassionate care of those living with HIV/AIDS. So, if those practising unprotected sexual intercourse with multiple partners were stigmatised, or even subject to statutory notification, they would not come forward for testing or palliative treatment. In addition, their partners would soon be stigmatised as well, regardless of whether or not they had multiple sexual partners. As Margaret Farley points out: 'stories abound . . . of the exile or even stoning of married women infected by their husbands, and of . . . women raped and infected by men who think that sex with virgins will prevent or cure their own infection by the AIDS virus'.[43] In any case, a more tolerant age today might move beyond discriminating against individuals because of their sexual behaviour. And even if it is still considered ethical to discriminate in this way, there may actually be little point in stigmatising individuals for their past behaviour once they have contracted the HIV virus. In addition, when it was supposed that the virus predominantly affected gay men, an understandable fear was raised of exacerbating homophobia in society at large (as has indeed has happened in parts of central Africa).

All of these are important points. As David Hollenbach was quoted as saying earlier: 'nothing said here should be taken to suggest otherwise'. Compassionate care of those living with HIV/AIDS is crucial for Christian ethics. Nevertheless, 'the virtue of tolerance [compassion], by itself, is not now a sufficient moral resource for addressing the problem [of the common good]'.[44] Again, as Margaret Farley points out: 'almost everyone agrees that some of the strategies necessary to prevent HIV/AIDS are actually available in most countries of the South – strategies such as reduction of the number of sexual partners, increased condom use, treatment of other sexually transmitted diseases, and safe injecting behaviour'.[45] Yet there is still a serious tension between these public health policies (especially if HIV/AIDS is treated as a deadly pandemic) and the compassionate care of individuals. There also remain serious tensions among Christians both about 'reduction of the number of sexual partners' and about 'increased condom use'. Some want to see not a 'reduction of the number of sexual partners' but complete abstinence outside exclusive monogamy. And Roman Catholic HIV/AIDS activists are themselves deeply divided about the permissibility of 'increased condom use' for the common good in order to reduce infection (as distinct from reducing conception). In society at large, the more urgent and drastic the pandemic is deemed to be, the more justifiable draconian public health measures may seem in the interests of the common good, and then the more seriously these measures may

---

[43] Farley, *Compassionate Respect*, pp. 10–11.   [44] Hollenbach, *Common Good*, p. 40.
[45] Farley, *Compassionate Respect*, pp. 9–10.

conflict with the compassionate care of individuals living with HIV/AIDS.

Over the last few years the *Journal of Medical Ethics* has discussed this tension – depicted here as the tension between the common good and the compassionate care of individuals – in a number of different areas. Anthony Pinching, a consultant immunologist with considerable clinical experience of patients living with HIV/AIDS, summarises the central dilemma as follows:

For clinicians, the most substantial tension has been in the potential or perceived conflict between the duty to the individual and the duty to protect others. How far should a doctor go in attempting to protect others from HIV risk from his patient? Many clinicians are very uncomfortable with knowing that an HIV-positive patient is continuing to have unsafe sex with a person whom the patient is unwilling to inform. After attempting to influence the patient's behaviour or willingness to disclose his HIV status, the clinician may be left either unable to act further because of confidentiality, or feeling obliged to breach confidentiality to protect the third party.[46]

Pinching's own inclination is not to breach patient confidentiality – on the prudential ground that such a breach to protect others will put at risk any further confidential information from patients – but he does not appear altogether comfortable with this position. After all, this particular HIV-positive patient knowingly puts another person seriously at risk without the latter's consent.

One set of subsequent articles puts this point sharply to the test by examining whether it would be right to criminalise knowing HIV transmission, even in a situation of consensual sex but without the HIV-positive status of the individual being disclosed. The tension here is deemed to be that 'there is a real danger that the criminalisation of HIV transmission may produce consequences that are not only morally unjustifiable but also unhelpful in terms of public health aims'.[47] A second set of articles discusses the ethical (common good) justification of seroprevalence monitoring of HIV in pregnant

---

[46] Anthony J. Pinching, Roger Higgs and Kenneth M. Boyd, 'The Impact of AIDS on Medical Ethics', *Journal of Medical Ethics*, 26:1 (2000), p. 5.

[47] Rebecca Bennett, Heather Draper and Lucy Firth, 'Ignorance is Bliss? HIV and Moral Duties and Legal Duties to Forewarn', *Journal of Medical Ethics*, 26:1 (2000), p. 15. See also, J. Chalmers, 'The Criminalisation of HIV Transmission', *Journal of Medical Ethics*, 28:3 (2002), pp. 160–3.

women by anonymised, unlinked testing. The author of one article here argues that such testing 'breaches the fundamental principles of respect for autonomy and beneficence if women are not informed of the advantages of named HIV testing' and that 'even with fully informed consent, for health professionals actively to request women to ignore the needs of third parties, and in particular of their unborn children, distorts the duty of care and undermines the goals of medicine'.[48] On this occasion, however, Pinching in his response argues that this 'seems to assume that doing things for the public good is somehow opposed to individual benefit'[49] and that it fails to distinguish between screening for research (which benefits many people) and clinical screening (which is for the benefit of that particular patient). Finally, another article evaluates the arguments for and against offering IVF to HIV discordant couples (where the male partner is HIV-positive and the female is not), raising acute questions about safety and public health particularly in relation to the potential offspring.[50]

It is tempting to use the Aristotelian principle cited earlier to resolve these ethical dilemmas, namely that 'the common good of the community should have primacy in setting direction for the lives of individuals, for it is a higher good than the particular goods of private persons'. But, as Hollenbach argues, establishing 'the common good of the community' needs careful and considered negotiation in a pluralistic society if tyrannous coercion is to be avoided. The rights of minorities can soon be overlooked when striving for 'the common good'. Just to take the final issue of discordant couples, there have been some very careful, and eventually successful, clinical decisions made allowing haemophiliac HIV-positive husbands to have their own children using a carefully monitored drug regime to minimise any possible harm to their wives or offspring.

It would take this book too far away from its task to examine each of these issues properly and then to resolve them. The central point to

[48] Paquita de Zulueta, 'The Ethics of Anonymised HIV Testing of Pregnant Women: a Reappraisal', *Journal of Medical Ethics*, 26:1 (2000), p. 21.

[49] Anthony J. Pinching, 'Commentary: the Ethics of Anonymised HIV Testing of Pregnant Women: a Reappraisal', *Journal of Medical Ethics*, 26:1 (2000), p. 24.

[50] M. Spriggs and T. Charles, 'Should HIV Discordant Couples Have Access to Assisted Reproductive Technologies?', *Journal of Medical Ethics*, 29:6 (2000), pp. 325–9.

note is that in several areas involving ethical responses to HIV/AIDS in the modern world there is a critical tension between the common good and the compassionate care of individuals. An adequate account of health care ethics should not ignore this tension.

More than that, this is a tension that can be found already in the wisdom present in the Synoptic healing stories. It was seen earlier in chapter 3 that the Synoptic Jesus shows anger towards the leper in Mark (1.43), anger towards the Pharisees in the story of the man with the withered hand (3.5), and in Matthew the two blind men are told 'sternly' by Jesus to tell no one (9.30). In other words, Jesus is depicted as both caring for the ill and disabled and caring about the prevalence of illness and disability. The passionate emotions depicted in the Synoptic healing stories appear sometimes to be directed at the disease itself or at the 'unclean spirits' and at other times at the faithlessness of the disciples or the religious authorities of the time. Compassionate care for the vulnerable goes hand in hand with passionate care about the conditions that make them vulnerable.

CHAPTER 6

Faith in health care ethics

Faith [*pistis*] is a very crucial and dominant feature of the Synoptic healing stories. Yet, as was also seen in chapter 3, there is considerable ambiguity about what exactly this 'faith' is. That chapter first showed that biblical commentators tend to disagree among themselves about the meaning of *pistis* in these stories and then it argued that the Synoptic stories themselves are inherently ambiguous. Three different levels of faith were detected in these stories: the first was faithful trust in Jesus as healer (demonstrated either by the persistent words or by the determined actions either of those who would be healed or of their family/friends); the second was faith as a mutual relationship between Jesus and those to be healed or their family/friends; the third was faith as a response to God. The present chapter will explore these three different levels of faith in the context of health care ethics today arguing that each is still surprisingly relevant.

For once it might be helpful to illustrate these three levels of faith from a healing story taken from the Fourth Gospel's account of Jesus healing an official's son (John 4.46–53) rather than from the Synoptic Gospels. After all, C. K. Barrett maintains that 'it seems very probable that the synoptic tradition (or a tradition very closely akin to it) lies immediately behind the Johannine narrative'.[1] There are indeed obvious parallels in this story with that of the healing of the centurion's servant (Matt. 8.5–13 / Luke 7.1–10). However, of all the healing

---

[1] C. K. Barrett, *The Gospel According to St John: an Introduction with Commentary and Notes on the Greek Text* (London: SPCK, 1967), p. 205.

stories in the Gospels, only the Johannine story unambiguously contains all three levels of faith:

4.46 There was a royal official whose son lay ill in Capernaum. 47 When he heard that Jesus had come from Judea to Galilee, he went and begged him to come down and heal his son, for he was at the point of death. 48 Then Jesus said to him, 'Unless you see signs and wonders you will not believe.' 49 The official said to him, 'Sir, come down before my little boy dies.' 50 Jesus said to him, 'Go, your son will live.' The man believed the word that Jesus spoke to him and started on his way. 51 As he was going down, his slaves met him and told him that his child was alive. 52 So he asked them the hour when he began to recover, and they said to him, 'Yesterday at one in the afternoon the fever left him.' 53 The father realised that this was the hour when Jesus had said to him, 'Your son will live.' So he himself believed, along with his whole household.

The first level of faith – faithful trust in Jesus as healer – does seem to be present in verse 50. Here the verb *pisteuein* is used with a dative noun: the official 'believes that what Jesus has said is true'.[2] Like the centurion in the Synoptic story, he shows an immediate faithful trust in Jesus' ability to heal at a distance. It was noted earlier that Matthew's story of the healing of the two blind men also refers unambiguously to this first level of faith, especially when Jesus asks the men: 'Do you believe [*pisteuete*] that I am able to do this?' (9.28). Mark's account of the woman with a haemorrhage, when compared with the parallel accounts of Matthew and Luke, also appears to focus upon this level. In Mark and Matthew (but not in Luke) the woman says before the healing: 'If I but touch his clothes, I will be made well' (Mark 5.28 / Matt. 9.21). And in Mark and Luke (but not in Matthew) Jesus' commendation of her faith ('Daughter, your faith has made you well') is delayed by a discussion about who touched him (Mark 5.30–3 / Luke 8.45–7). With both of these features in his account Mark seems particularly to emphasise the unilateral character of the woman's faithful trust, even if it eventually becomes more mutual with Jesus' final response.

The second level of faith – faith as a mutual relationship between Jesus and those to be healed or their family/friends – shapes the Johannine story. As in the Synoptic story of the Syro-Phoenician

---

[2] Barrett, *St John*, p. 207.

woman (Mark 7.24–30 / Matt. 15.21–8), the parent comes to Jesus and begs him to heal his child, Jesus probes, the parent responds, and then Jesus proclaims the healing. In John *pisteuein* is used in Jesus' probe (4.48): in Matthew Jesus exclaims at the end 'Woman, great is your faith!' (15.28). Again it was noted earlier that 'mutuality' in some form does seem to differentiate the tenth leper's response from that of the other nine in Luke's puzzling story of the ten lepers (17.11–19). He uses the commendation 'your faith has made you well' once more here, but only for the tenth leper. At a negative level, in Mark and Matthew there is also the incident in Jesus' hometown when an absence of faith/mutuality was associated with comparatively little healing. Mark, having noted Jesus' inability to do much healing there, concludes simply that 'he was amazed at their unbelief [*apistian*]' (6.6). Matthew summarises the situation with a direct causal connection: 'And he did not do many deeds of power there, because of their unbelief' (13.58).

The third level of faith – faith as a response to God – comes at the end of the story. In verse 53, unlike in verse 50, the verb *pisteuein* is used absolutely. For John this seems to mean simply that 'he became a Christian',[3] as it does in the Prologue (1.7 'so that all might believe through him') and in two out of three of the other Johannine healing stories. So at the end of the story of the healing of the blind man, the one healed exclaims 'Lord, I believe' (9.38) and proceeds to worship Jesus, and the story of the raising of Lazarus concludes with the verse: 'Many of the Jews therefore, who had come with Mary and had seen what Jesus did, believed in him' (11.45). Most striking of all is the exchange between Jesus and Martha just before the raising of Lazarus:

> Jesus said to her, 'I am the resurrection and the life. Those who believe in me, even though they die, will live, and everyone who lives and believes in me will never die. Do you believe this?' She said to him, 'Yes, Lord, I believe that you are the Messiah, the Son of God, the one coming into the world.' (11.25–7)

Such high Christology cannot be matched in the Synoptic Gospels' healing stories. In the latter this third level of faith appears

---

[3] Barrett, *St John*, p. 207.

more elliptically (as seen earlier) in Jesus' response to his disciples after the healing of the epileptic boy in Mark: 'This kind cannot be driven out by anything but prayer' (9.29). Or in people glorifying God after a healing, as in the dramatic end to the healing of the paralytic in Mark: 'And he stood up, and immediately took the mat and went out before all of them; so that they were all amazed and glorified God, saying, "We have never seen anything like this!"' (2.12), and especially in Matthew's added comment that 'they glorified God, who had given such authority to men' (9.7).

TWO SECULAR ACCOUNTS OF FAITH

Following the pattern set in these Synoptic healing stories, it is possible that without at least some trust in the medical professional (First-Level Faith) – or, better, a mutual confidence between patient and professional (Second-Level Faith) – then healing may well be imperilled. Faith in the form of trust (but not always mutual confidence), and often in the form of implicit religious commitment (Third-Level Faith), was characteristically present in the paternalistic medical practice (itself dependent upon patient compliance) of a previous generation. Today this has radically changed. Two non-religious academics have been particularly successful in articulating the problem that this poses for modern health care. The most recent of these is the philosopher Onora O'Neill, notably in her influential Reith and Gifford Lectures. She argues that, within a medical context that can now be too dominated by an excessively individualistic concept of patient autonomy together with a mechanical approach to institutional audit, this trust has been weakened. In contrast, a healing relationship understood in terms of mutual confidence offers a model of faith (Second-Level Faith) that respects both patient and professional autonomies and seeks to relate the two to each other. A generation earlier, the sociologist Paul Halmos' influential book *The Faith of the Counsellors* made an even stronger argument. Having noted that secular counsellors tend to depict their role in 'scientific' terms and, in the process, ignore value-commitments that are also fundamental to good counselling, he argued that it is the Judaeo-Christian virtue of love/*agape* that is the usually unacknowledged, but essential, ingredient of effective counselling (Third-Level Faith).

In her Gifford Lectures O'Neill traces the way that a highly individualistic understanding of autonomy has become dominant in health care ethics, but argues that this has created a sharp paradox:

We might expect the increasing attention paid to individual rights and to autonomy to have increased public trust in the ways in which medicine, science and biotechnology are practised and regulated. Greater rights and autonomy give individuals greater control over the ways they live and increase their capacities to resist others' demands and institutional pressures. Yet amid widespread and energetic efforts to respect persons and their autonomy and to improve regulatory structures, public trust in medicine, science and biotechnology has seemingly faltered.[4]

She is aware that some would attribute this loss of trust to the biosciences becoming increasingly complex, remote and risky. But she is not convinced, since 'traditional hazards such as endemic tuberculosis or contaminated water supplies, food scarcity and fuel poverty were neither minimal nor controllable by those at risk from them in the recent past, and are neither minimal nor controllable for those who still face them in poorer societies today'.[5] It simply is not the fact that those living in the modern, Western world face a riskier and more hazardous environment than either their ancestors or their contemporaries in the South. On the contrary, they live longer and enjoy much better health. Yet, so she argues, they are increasingly losing trust in medical (and scientific) professionals, and, ironically, putting increasing trust in alternative 'therapies':

where people perceive others as untrustworthy they may place their trust capriciously and anxiously, veering between trusting qualified doctors and trusting unregulated alternative practitioners, between trusting scientific claims and trusting those alternative, greenish or counter-cultural campaigners, or modish therapies and diets, between trusting established technologies and medicines and trusting untested or exotic technologies and products.[6]

O'Neill places a large part of the blame for this situation on two powerful social agendas – the audit agenda and the openness

---

[4] Onora O'Neill, *Autonomy and Trust in Bioethics* (Cambridge: Cambridge University Press, 2002), p. 3.

[5] O'Neill, *Autonomy and Trust in Bioethics*, p. 8.

[6] O'Neill, *Autonomy and Trust in Bioethics*, p. 12.

agenda – that have been extensively deployed over the last twenty years in order to improve accountability, and with it trustworthiness, in many areas of public life. She believes that in reality they have tended to reduce public trust. Of course she faces an obvious problem here: the sentence just quoted at the end of the previous paragraph contrasts 'qualified doctors' with 'unregulated alternative practitioners', 'scientific claims' with 'modish therapies and diets', and 'established technologies and medicines' with those that are 'untested'. These very contrasts depend upon audited and regulated qualifications and claims. However, she maintains that there has been a radical change of scale and location in the new social agendas:

The older systems were typically *qualitative*, often *internal* and *local*; they depended on high levels of *trust* and permitted institutions considerable *individual autonomy*; they looked at the *primary activities* of institutions in *real time*. In contrast, the new systems are *quantitative*, are *external* and often conducted at *arm's length*; they manifest *low trust* of those being called to account and exert considerable *discipline*; they look at *systems* and are typically conducted *retrospectively*.[7]

The new systems, intended to restore trust in modern society, in reality foster public suspicion and a decrease in public trust.

In her Reith Lectures O'Neill is even more forceful:

In the end, the new culture of accountability provides incentives for arbitrary and unprofessional choices. Lecturers may publish prematurely because their department's research rating and its funding requires it. Schools may promote certain subjects in which it is easier to get 'As' in public examinations in those subjects. Hospital trusts have to focus on waiting lists even where these are not the most significant measures of medical quality. To add to their grief, the Sisyphean task of pushing institutional performance up the league tables is made harder by constantly redefining and adding targets and introducing initiatives, and of course with no account taken of the costs of competing for initiative funding. In the New World of accountability, conscientious professionals often find that the public claim to mistrust them – but the public still demand their services … The pursuit of ever more perfect accountability provides citizens and consumers, patients and parents with more information, more comparisons more complaints systems; but it also builds a culture of suspicion, low morale

[7] O'Neill, *Autonomy and Trust in Bioethics*, p. 132. She is using the theory of Michael Power here (see his *The Audit Society*, Oxford: Oxford University Press, 1996).

and may ultimately lead to professional cynicism, and then we would have grounds for public mistrust. Perhaps the present revolution in accountability will make us all trustworthier. Perhaps we shall be trusted once again. But I think that this is a vain hope – not because accountability is undesirable or unnecessary, but because currently fashionable methods of accountability damage rather than repair trust.[8]

Yet her remedy of 'intelligent accountability' is, in the end, remarkably thin:

Intelligent accountability, I suspect, requires more attention to good governance and fewer fantasies about total control. Good governance is possible only if institutions are allowed some margin for self-governance of a form appropriate to their particular tasks, within a framework of financial and other reporting.[9]

She does, however, provide a rather thicker account of autonomy. Together with Gordon Stirrat I have argued elsewhere[10] that this account is a very important contribution to health care ethics. O'Neill argues at length that the dominant notion of 'autonomy' in health care ethics has become too individualistic. She reminds us that Mill 'hardly ever uses the word, autonomy' and when he does so refers to states rather than individuals. 'Mill's version of autonomy', she asserts, 'sees individuals not merely as choosing to implement whatever desires they happen to have at a given moment, but as taking charge of those desires, as reflecting on and selecting among them in distinctive ways.' She also maintains that Kant never speaks of autonomous persons or individuals and 'he does not equate it with any distinctive form of personal independence or self-expression . . . Kantian autonomy is manifested in a life in which duties are met, in which there is a respect for others and their rights'. His view of autonomy is not 'a form of self expression', but 'rather a matter of acting on certain sorts of principles, and specifically on principles of obligation . . . there can be no possibility of freedom for any one individual if that person acts without reference to all other moral agents'.[11]

[8] Lecture 3.3–4: www.bbc.co.uk/radio4/reith2002.
[9] Lecture 3.4: www.bbc.co.uk/radio4/reith2002.
[10] Gordon M. Stirrat and Robin Gill, 'Autonomy in Medical Ethics After O'Neill', *Journal of Medical Ethics*, 31:2 (2005), pp. 127–30.
[11] O'Neill, *Autonomy and Trust in Bioethics*, pp. 83–5.

O'Neill entitles this 'principled autonomy': unlike individualistic accounts of autonomy it crucially contains a notion of mutuality. The contrast between these two understandings of 'autonomy' in health care ethics is strikingly illustrated in a recent edition of the *Journal of Medical Ethics*. In her article in this, O'Neill argues again that 'contemporary accounts of autonomy have lost touch with their Kantian origins, in which the links between autonomy and respect for persons are well argued'.[12] Five pages later John Harris claims (the next chapter will inspect this further) that:

Autonomy, the values expressed as the ability to choose and have the freedom to choose between competing conceptions of how to live and indeed of why we do so, is connected to individuality in that *it is only by the exercise of autonomy that our lives become in any sense our own* [my italics]. By shaping our lives for ourselves we assert our own values and our individuality.[13]

Despite being a Gifford Lecturer, O'Neill seldom refers to religious issues (and such references as she does make are usually negative) and prefers the term 'trust' to 'faith'. Writing a generation earlier, Paul Halmos quite deliberately wrote about the 'faith' of counsellors. The central argument of his book *The Faith of the Counsellors*[14] is that secular counsellors go to extraordinary lengths to disguise the fact that altruistic love – embedded in society through centuries of Christian socialisation – is an essential axiom of their work. Despite many layers of 'scientific' jargon and despite denials by secular counsellors that their work is religiously motivated or shaped, Halmos argued that it makes little sense if the role of Christian *agape* is excluded. He was not, of course, arguing that counsellors themselves needed to become Christians to do their work effectively (or even truthfully), but he was convinced that secular scholars should acknowledge this religious heritage more clearly than they generally do.

This difference between O'Neill and Halmos is instructive. As already noted, in the 1960s when Halmos was writing, health care ethics in Britain (and in the United States) was still dominated by

---

[12] Onora O'Neill, 'Some Limits of Informed Consent', *Journal of Medical Ethics*, 29:1 (2003), p. 5.
[13] John Harris, 'Consent and End of Life Decisions', *Journal of Medical Ethics*, 29:1 (2003), pp. 10–11.
[14] Paul Halmos, *The Faith of the Counsellors* (London: Constable, 1965).

theologians, church leaders and hospital chaplains. In contrast, O'Neill is writing at a time when philosophers and lawyers are dominant in health care ethics. In the earlier context it would have been far more natural to assume that *agape* and *pistis* were essential ingredients of health care ethics (even if their biblical or metaphysical roots were played down). In the later context O'Neill is simply puzzled that 'autonomy' is now understood so individualistically and that 'trust' is in decline. Turning on the messenger, she blames the new audit culture. But perhaps Charles Taylor is nearer the mark. Once again, it may be the growing gap between personal resonance and a shared understanding of cosmic order that is the more serious problem here. In the generation between Halmos and O'Neill, medical professionals themselves appear to have shifted from an implicitly shared culture (based roughly upon Judaeo-Christian assumptions) to a pluralistic culture largely lacking a shared understanding of cosmic order. Some doctors will now have come to share the secularist assumptions so prevalent in the universities in which they trained. Others increasingly come from Islamic, Hindu, Sikh or Buddhist cultures. Judaeo-Christian values – once shared broadly by the religiously active and non-religious Humanists alike – have inevitably become socially contentious. So it may not be too surprising both that philosophers and lawyers have become so dominant in health care ethics and, now that they have, that 'softer' notions of mutuality, altruism and trust (with their deep religious roots) have become more marginal. Inevitably philosophers want conceptual clarity and lawyers want clear processes of enforceability. In contrast, mutuality, altruism and trust need to be engendered and nurtured within communities. And perhaps it is communities moulded by abiding religious traditions that are particularly effective in achieving this. Or, to express this differently, it could be that it is Third-Level Faith that is able to give particular substance to First- and Second-Level Faith.

The pioneer sociologist Emile Durkheim certainly would have assumed as much. Although a secularist himself, he argued that altruism in particular was derived from, and supported by, religious belief and ritual. In his early study of suicide he identified 'altruistic suicide' as a particular form of suicide that was characteristic of the religiously motivated. Undoubtedly he would have seen the perpetrators of September 11 and the numerous suicide bombers in Iraq and elsewhere in the Middle East today as clear examples of this. In his mature work *The Elementary Forms of the Religious Life* he explained how a flag in battle could become a religious totem, itself standing for the altruism demanded of soldiers in time of war:

It is to this that we connect the emotions it excites. It is this which is loved, feared, respected; it is to this that we are grateful; it is for this that we sacrifice ourselves. The soldier who dies for the flag, dies for his country; but as a matter of fact, in his own consciousness, it is the flag that has taken the first place. It sometimes happens that this even directly determines action. Whether one isolated standard remains in the hands of the enemy or not does not determine the fate of the country, yet the soldier allows himself to be killed to regain it.[15]

The connections between totem, religion, morality, community and country were foundational to Durkheim's sociology of religion. Each was intimately connected with the others. For him religion was essentially communal and it was religious/communal rites, totems and beliefs that inspired individuals to move beyond egotism and to become altruistic:

However complex the outward manifestations of the religious life may be, at bottom it is one and simple. It responds everywhere to one and the same need, and is everywhere derived from one and the same mental state. In all its forms, its object is to raise man above himself and to make him lead a life superior to that which he would lead, if he followed only his own individual whims: beliefs express this life in representations; rites organize and regulate its working.[16]

For Durkheim it was religion that enabled people to be altruistic and to lead a more 'superior' life ... in other words to raise individuals above themselves and their self-centred whims. Of course Durkheim had a very functional understanding of 'religion' and for him 'religion' and 'community' were all but tautologies. Famously he concluded that 'the old gods are growing old or already dead, and others are not yet born', but then immediately added:

But this state of incertitude and confused agitation cannot last for ever. A day will come when our societies will know again those hours of creative effervescence, in the course of which new ideas arise and new formulae are found which serve for a while as a guide to humanity.[17]

[15] Emile Durkheim, *The Elementary Forms of the Religious Life* [1915], (London: George Allen and Unwin, 1976), p. 220.
[16] Durkheim, *Elementary Forms*, p. 414.   [17] Durkheim, *Elementary Forms*, pp. 427–8.

RELIGION AND HEALTH CARE

Interestingly there does seem to be growing empirical evidence that there is a connection between religious belonging and health. This suggests that religious belonging is a significant (but often ignored) independent variable in promoting physical and psychological health. It is possible that people with strong religious affiliations are more likely than others to have a sense of purpose in life and to be altruistic (as shown earlier in *Churchgoing and Christian Ethics*). In turn, such motivation may have important implications for physical and psychological health.

The work of the physician Harold Koenig, of Duke University Medical Center, and of the social scientist Byron Johnson, of the Center for Research on Religion and Urban Civil Society at the University of Pennsylvania, has been particularly important for marshalling this empirical evidence about Third-Level Faith. Koenig has directed and coordinated a range of empirical studies[18] and co-written the principal textbook in this area,[19] while Johnson has provided a systematic review of American and European empirical studies.[20] Together their work provides a very strong case for claiming that religious faith/belonging has an effect upon mortality and morbidity.

Well aware of the methodological criticisms of some of the earlier empirical studies of religion and health,[21] Koenig has recently summarised the research achieved as follows:

During the twentieth century more than twelve hundred studies examined the relationship between religion and health, with the majority finding a significant positive association. Many of these were cross-sectional studies

---

[18] E.g. Harold G. Koenig, Judith C. Hayes, David B. Larson, Linda K. George, Harvey Jay Cohen, Michael E. McCullough, Keith G. Meador and Dan G. Blazer, 'Does Religious Attendance Prolong Survival? A Six-Year Follow-up Study of 3,968 Older Adults', *Journal of Gerontology: Medical Sciences*, 54 A:7 (1999), M370–M376.

[19] Harold G. Koenig, Michael E. McCullough and David B. Larson, *Handbook of Religion and Health* (New York: Oxford University Press, 2001).

[20] Byron R. Johnson, Ralph Brett Tompkins and Derek Webb, *Objective Hope: Assessing the Effectiveness of Faith-Based Organizations: a Review of the Literature* (Philadelphia: Center for Research on Religion and Urban Civil Society, University of Pennsylvania, 2001 [www.crrucs.org]).

[21] See R. P. Sloan, E. Bagiella and T. Powell, 'Viewpoint: Religion, Spirituality and Medicine', *The Lancet*, 353 (1999), pp. 664–7.

and weak in terms of methodology. There were also, however, many well-designed prospective studies, and even a handful of clinical trials that verified and supported the findings from the cross-sectional studies.[22]

He then reviews these findings under six broad headings, reaching the conclusion that 'there is growing evidence from systematic research that religious beliefs and practices are related to better mental health, better physical health, and less need for health services', even though he admits that 'we know that religious and spiritual involvement does not *always* have positive effects on health, and even when it does so, the underlying biological mechanisms are poorly understood':[23]

Coping and depression. Hospitalized medically ill patients who rely on religion cope better than those who do not. Patients who depend on religion are less likely to develop depression, and even if they do become depressed, they recover more quickly from depression than do patients who are less religious. This is also true for caregivers of patients with Alzheimer's disease or cancer, who appeared to adapt more quickly to the caregiver role if more religious . . .

Suicide and substance abuse. There is even more consensus when rates of suicide and substance abuse are considered. Of 68 studies examining suicide, 84% found lower rates of suicide or more negative attitudes toward it among the more religious. Of the nearly 140 studies that have examined religious involvement and abuse of alcohol or drugs, 90% found a statistically significant inverse correlation between the two . . .

Positive emotions. Well-being and positive emotions such as joy, hope, and optimism also appear to be disproportionately prevalent among the religious. Of 100 studies in the past century that examined these relationships, 79 found that religious persons had significantly greater well-being, life satisfaction, or happiness than did those who were less religious . . .

Social support. Almost all studies examining religion and social support find a significant correlation (19 of 20 studies). Not only does the religious person have a larger support network, but the quality of that social network is higher and may be more durable than secular sources of support when chronic illness strikes . . .

Physical health. There is mounting evidence from the field of psychoneuroimmunology that positive emotions and social support are associated

[22] Harold G. Koenig, *Spirituality in Patient Care* (Philadelphia and London: Templeton Foundation Press, 2002), p. 8.
[23] Koenig, *Spirituality in Patient Care*, p. 13.

with better immune functioning and more robust cardiovascular health, and that the corollary also appears to be true, i.e., that depression and social isolation worsen health and slow recovery from illness ... In fact, there is a consistent relationship between degree of religious involvement and lower mortality ... twelve of the thirteen most recent studies using the best research methodology found longer survival among the more religious. This finding is particularly robust in terms of religious community involvement. The difference in survival between those who attend religious services weekly or more and those who do not attend is approximately seven years ...

Need for health services. Research suggests that religious persons spend less time in the hospital, perhaps because they are healthier and have more support within the community ... In terms of actual number of days hospitalised, patients attending religious services at least several times per month were hospitalised an average of six days in the previous year, compared to twelve days for those attending services only a few times per year or not at all.[24]

All of this suggests that well-being, life-satisfaction, community and abiding support networks are stronger among the religiously active than among those who are not religiously active, and that the physical and mental health (with corresponding better mortality rates) of the former is better than the latter. If all of this is so it does suggest that Durkheim's broad sociological claims were not misplaced. He was only half-correct, though, in predicting that 'a day will come when our societies will know again those hours of creative effervescence, in the course of which new ideas arise and new formulae are found which serve for a while as a guide to humanity'. As José Casanova has pointed out, it may actually be older forms of religion that still act as guides even within the modern world.[25]

Byron Johnson, together with his two research assistants, has built upon Harold Koenig's massive marshalling of research and clinical data, refined and systematised it, added extra dimensions of health and well-being, and compared it with evidence about the social effectiveness of faith-based organisations. The results are impressive, not least because Johnson is cautious about making strong empirically based claims about the social effectiveness of faith-based organisations. And this

[24] Koenig, *Spirituality in Patient Care*, pp. 8–12.
[25] José Casanova, 'Beyond European and American Exceptionalisms', in Grace Davie, Paul Heelas and Linda Woodhead (eds.), *Predicting Religion: Christian, Secular and Alternative Futures* (Aldershot, Hants: Ashgate, 2003).

despite one of the remits of the Center for Research on Religion and Urban Civil Society being to focus on 'how national and local faith-based organizations help to solve big-city social problems'. Having located and analysed 25 studies that examined the effectiveness of faith-based organisations (23 of which concluded that faith-based interventions – for example, among prisoners or drug addicts – had been beneficial), he reaches the conclusion that his review 'has uncovered a number of solid case studies and multivariate evaluations providing at least preliminary evidence that faith-based programs can provide effective interventions', but then adds immediately that 'it is important to note, however, that the small number of intentional studies reviewed by itself, cannot unequivocally certify the claim that faith-based programs are more effective than their secular counterparts'.[26]

However, when he reviews the research on the health and well-being of individuals, he is much less cautious about the social significance of religion. Having analysed 669 studies in this area he reaches two much stronger conclusions:

(1) research on religious practices and health outcomes indicates that higher levels of religious involvement are associated with: reduced hypertension, longer survival, less depression, lower levels of drug and alcohol use and abuse, less promiscuous sexual behaviors, reduced likelihood of suicide, lower rates of delinquency among youth, and reduced criminal activity among adults. This review provides overwhelming evidence that higher levels of religious involvement and practices make for an important protective factor that buffers or insulates individuals from deleterious outcomes.

(2) research on religious practices and various measures of well-being reveals higher levels of religious involvement are associated with increased levels of: well-being, hope, purpose, meaning in life, and educational attainment. This review of organic religion documents that religious commitment or practices make for an important factor promoting an array of prosocial behaviors and thus enhancing various beneficial outcomes.[27]

Of course it is tempting to jump from this evidence about the health and well-being of religiously active individuals (what Johnson terms 'organic religion') to conclusions, for example, about the

---

[26] Johnson et al., *Objective Hope*, p. 21.   [27] Johnson et al., *Objective Hope*, p. 7.

effectiveness of faith-based interventions in prisons (he terms this 'intentional religion'). However, Johnson avoids making this jump, arguing instead that better research is needed in this second area.

He is, though, in little doubt about the overall social significance of organic religion. In each of the areas of health and well-being analysed the beneficial effects of religious involvement were highly significant (and harmful outcomes minimal). So, 76% of the studies analysed found that religious involvement was linked with reduced levels of hypertension; 75% with greater longevity; 68% with less depression; 87% with lower levels of drug, and 94% with lower levels of alcohol, use/abuse; 97% with less sexual promiscuity; 87% with reduced likelihood of suicide; and 78% with lower rates of delinquency and criminal activity. Similarly, 81% of the studies analysed found that religious involvement was linked with greater 'happiness, life satisfaction, morale, positive affect or some other measure of well-being'; 83% with 'having hope or a sense of purpose or meaning in life', as well as with increased social support; 65% with increases in self-esteem; and 84% with improved educational attainment.

Johnson concludes that 'this review of a large number of diverse studies leaves one with the observation that, in general, the effect of religion on physical and mental health outcomes is remarkably positive'. Nevertheless, he still points out that 'more research utilizing longitudinal and experimental designs is needed to further address important causal linkages between organic religion and myriad social and behavioural outcomes'.[28]

His caution is wise given the methodological criticism that has sometimes been made of this genre of research. A central problem is that an expensive research project on religious involvement and health/well-being is unlikely to attract public funds. From a public health perspective in a pluralistic society there is, after all, little prospect of being able to link such a project directly to public social policy. Having made strong methodological criticisms of the research in this area as it was in 1999, Richard Sloan and his colleagues point out the obvious ethical problems of making such a direct link to public policy. They argue that 'when doctors depart from areas of established expertise to promote a non-medical agenda,

---

[28] Johnson et al., *Objective Hope*, p. 15.

they abuse their status as professionals . . . we question inquiries into a patient's spiritual life in the services of making recommendations that link religious practice with better health outcomes'.[29] To reinforce this point, they suggest that it would be just as inappropriate for doctors to advise the unmarried to marry on the grounds that marriage is also associated with lower mortality. In any case, they insist, 'since all human beings, devout or profane, ultimately will succumb to illness, we wish to avoid the additional burden or guilt for moral failure to those whose physical health fails before our own'.[30]

There is also a very obvious theological objection to making a direct link between such research on religious involvement and public health policy. From a theological perspective, it suggests a distinctly instrumental understanding of Third-Level Faith – as a commodity that is simply beneficial for health. This point needs to be addressed very soon.

Without such a link, funding for research in this area is likely to remain precarious and research projects, as a result, may well remain rather varied in quality. Large, longitudinal, randomised and scientifically stratified samples are likely to remain exceptions amid enthusiastic, but more amateur, research projects. In the data for my own *Churchgoing and Christian Ethics* I was very fortunate in having direct access to two extensive and highly professional sources, the longitudinal *British Household Panel Survey* and the extensive *British Social Attitudes*. It would be extremely expensive for any individual researcher to replicate such national data. However, the data came with a price: I could only use data from questions that other people had devised for their own purposes. Inevitably this is frustrating and limiting. Harold Koenig has been assisted by the Templeton Foundation, and Byron Johnson by the Pew Charitable Trusts, to fund their considerable marshalling of research studies. Nevertheless, this is unlikely to become an area of health study research which commands the sort of funds that would make possible incontrovertible evidence using nationally representative samples.

---

[29] Sloan, Bagiella and Powell, 'Viewpoint: Religion, Spirituality and Medicine', p. 666.
[30] Sloan, Bagiella and Powell, 'Viewpoint: Religion, Spirituality and Medicine', p. 666.

However, there are some important exceptions. To take a single striking example, the demographer Robert Hummer and his colleagues showed how the very large and professional American *National Health Interview Survey* could be exploited to assess a possible connection between differing rates of churchgoing and adult mortality. The 1987 supplement of this survey, the Cancer Risk Factor Supplement-Epidemiological Study (with a useable sample size of 21,204 people that could be linked to follow-up data in 1995, at which time almost one in ten had died), asks a question about frequency of religious attendance, alongside many other socio-demographic variables. In this respect it is very close to the data that I exploit myself in *Churchgoing and Christian Ethics*. Unlike many other surveys that have a variety of different ways of assessing 'religious involvement' (ranging from affiliation, to membership, to 'religiosity'), this particular source focuses upon frequency of attendance (measured on a four-point scale ranging from religious attendance 'never' to 'more than once a week'). I have argued extensively elsewhere that it is indeed religious attendance that is the most useful and reliable variable of religious involvement when synchronic and diachronic comparisons are made.[31]

Hummer et al. note that, compared with numerous socio-economic mortality studies, those concerned with religious involvement are few, and none, until this study, 'analyzed a nationally representative sample across the entire adult age range; none looked at life expectancy differences across levels of religious involvement; some date back several decades; and few included an extensive array of independent variables or analyzed cause-of-death differences by religious involvement'.[32] Four questions guided this new study: (1) Is religious involvement associated with US adult mortality? (2) If so, to what extent and why? (3) Does the association vary across social and demographic characteristics? (4) Does the association vary by underlying cause of death? In summary form, Hummer et al. find that religious (increased) involvement is clearly associated with US adult mortality, that it does significantly improve life expectancy,

---

[31] See my *The 'Empty' Church Revisited* (Aldershot, Hants: Ashgate, 2003), chapter 1.
[32] Robert A. Hummer, Richard G. Rogers, Charles B. Nam and Christopher G. Ellison, 'Religious Involvement and US Adult Mortality', *Demography*, 36:2 (1999), p. 274.

and that, although other socio-demographic characteristics and different underlying causes of death are also significant, religious involvement still remains a significant variable once they are taken into consideration. The overall findings run directly counter to the 'sense among much of the scientific community that religious effects are minor at best or are even irrelevant'.[33]

Using a variety of multivariate models of religious attendance and mortality, Hummer et al. take into account such factors as the higher age, socio-economic status and (possibly) more robust health of churchgoers. Clearly if these are not taken properly into account non-churchgoers might, in reality, simply consist of those who are too ill to go to church or of low socio-economic-status men who are normally under-represented among churchgoers. They also take into account such mediating factors as the lower levels of smoking and drinking among churchgoers,[34] the stronger social support among churchgoers, and their more stable marriages. They also look carefully at variation across groups (such as ethnicity) and variation in the cause of death. At a straightforward descriptive level (using life expectancy estimates aged 20), they find that 'for the overall population, the life expectancy gap between those who attend [church/temple] more than once a week (62.9) and those who never attend (55.3) is over seven years, similar to the female-male and white-black gaps in US life expectancy ... (and) among blacks, most strikingly, there is nearly a 14-year advantage'.[35] Controlling for age, sex and race, religious attendance still remains significant: 'compared with those who attend more than once a week, those who never attend exhibit 87% higher risks of dying'. Controlling for such factors as smoking and drinking does reduce this, but those who never attend still show 'substantially higher mortality than those who attend more often'.[36] Social ties again reduce this difference but do not eliminate it, but socio-economic factors (surprisingly) do not reduce it. All of the different causes of death are significantly related to religious attendance, but some (such as respiratory diseases, diabetes and

[33] Hummer et al., 'Religious Involvement and US Adult Mortality', p. 283.
[34] For this see also my *Churchgoing and Christian Ethics*, pp. 167f.
[35] Hummer et al., 'Religious Involvement and US Adult Mortality', p. 277–8.
[36] Hummer et al., 'Religious Involvement and US Adult Mortality', p. 278.

infectious diseases) are more strongly related than others (such as
accidents, circulatory diseases and cancer). The never-attenders are
almost four times more likely than the most frequent attenders to die
from the first set of diseases (mediating life-style factors appear
particularly important here).

In short Hummer et al. conclude that, even if the causal linkages
are still not properly understood, 'a strong association between
infrequent or no religious attendance and higher mortality risk
persisted for overall mortality and most causes of death even after
we controlled for all of the independent variables'.[37] Given the
quality of the data-set here, this an important finding.

FAITH IN THE PUBLIC DOMAIN

But does this empirical evidence have a significant contribution to
make to health care ethics today in the public forum of a Western,
pluralistic society? My remit is not to focus exclusively upon the
Christian community – within *that* the combined efforts of Koenig,
Johnson and Hummer et al. may well be comforting – but rather to
be concerned with society at large. Even if the religiously inactive, let
alone those actively hostile to religion, could be convinced that
religious involvement has significant health benefits, what ethical
implications might they be able to draw from this?

One response to this question is to point instead to the harmful
effects of religion.[38] Koenig devotes a chapter to this topic in his
Spirituality in Patient Care, admitting that religion has indeed at
times been used to justify hatred, aggression and guilt:

Equally as worrisome, religion may be used *instead* of medical care.
Members of certain fundamentalist religious sects may fail to seek prenatal
or obstetric care on religious grounds, greatly increasing the risk of infant
and maternal mortality ... Active resistance against childhood vaccination
occurs in a number of religious groups around the world and has resulted in
recent outbreaks of polio, rubella, whooping cough, and other infectious

---

[37] Hummer et al., 'Religious Involvement and US Adult Mortality', p. 283.
[38] For example see Lawrence Osborn and Andrew Walker (eds.), *Harmful Religion: an
Exploration of Religious Abuse* (London: SPCK 1997), and Neale Krause and Keith M.
Wulff, 'Religious Doubt and Health: Exploring the Potential Dark Side of Religion',
Sociology of Religion, 65:1 (2004), pp. 35–56.

diseases. Life-saving treatments may be avoided or discontinued on religious grounds. Patients may stop their medications after attending a healing service in order to 'demonstrate their faith'.[39]

In Britain, it has been claimed that a young woman died after stopping her medication as a result of Morris Cerullo's 1992 Mission to London.[40]

For this and other reasons, subsequent Cerullo missions were extensively lobbied by disability groups and by the Anglican general practitioner Peter May.

However, Koenig argues that such cases are comparatively uncommon. Citing one report[41] that 172 children died in the United States between 1975 and 1995 as a result of parents withholding medical treatment on religious grounds, he calculates that 83% of these cases came from five marginal, sectarian groups. In Britain, too, it is probably remarkable that, despite considerable media scrutiny at the time, only one death *was* attributed directly to the Morris Cerullo missions. It will also be the experience of many who have served on local hospital or trust medical ethics committees that a disproportionate amount of time can be spent on comparatively rare cases of Jehovah's Witnesses refusing life-sustaining blood transfusions. While it is widely recognised that this can happen – and that it can involve acute ethical dilemmas about properly informed consent (especially if a Jehovah's Witness pastor, elder, partner or even elderly parent is present when this consent is sought) – it hardly represents an everyday experience.

Nevertheless, a point remains that Koenig may underestimate. If religious opposition to hormonal and barrier contraception in the present, or to anaesthetics in the past, is also identified as 'harmful', then the harmful effects of religion on health would be considerably more extensive. As noted earlier, the symposium *Religion, Health and Suffering* does have some justification in concluding that 'religions have not always been the caring forces their adherents sometimes

---

[39] Koenig, *Spirituality in Patient Care*, pp. 78–9.
[40] See Nancy A. Schaefer, 'Making the Rulers Tremble!: Morris Cerullo World Evangelism's 1994 Mission to London Revival', in Marion Bowman (ed.), *Healing and Religion* (Enfield Lock, Middlesex: Hisarlik Press, 2000), p. 24.
[41] S. Asser and R. Swan, 'Child Fatalities from Religious-Motivated Medical Neglect', *Pediatrics*, 101 (1998), pp. 625–9.

emphasise'.[42] And if the harmful effects of religion are examined more widely beyond health issues, then considerable caution is needed. William Schweiker has argued at length that Christian ethicists today do need to acknowledge frankly that some forms of Christian theology have contributed harmfully to an increasingly globalised world – for example, by fostering ecological degradation or by energising inter-religious or intra-religious wars.[43]

Koenig emphasises that 'the key to handling situations where religious beliefs conflict with medical or psychiatric care is for the physician to enter into the worldview of the patient and attempt to understand the logic of the decision'.[44] In a globalised society this is especially important. Second-Level Faith, as a mutual relationship between healer and the one to be healed, does seem to demand this. Sloan, Bagiella and Powell, too, believe that 'a thorough understanding of a patient's religious values can be extremely important in discussing critical medical issues, such as care at the end of life … irrespective of the practitioner's religion, respectful attention must be paid to the impact of religion on the patient's decisions about health care'.[45]

Yet there is still a crucial difference between Koenig and Sloan, Bagiella and Powell. Koenig is finally not convinced by the latter's ethical arguments about the danger of upsetting patients and inducing guilt by enquiring into their religious commitments [Third-Level Faith]. He argues that, provided this is done sensitively and respectfully, 'physicians inquire into many personal aspects of patients' lives because those areas affect the patient's health or medical care … (they) do not devalue patients who are single, without friends, or who are poor, but they do need to know about these conditions because of the potential relationship to health and the kind of support

---

[42] John R. Hinnells and Roy Porter (eds.), *Religion, Health and Suffering* (London and New York: Kegan Paul International, 1999), p. xi.

[43] William Schweiker, *Theological Ethics and Global Dynamics: In the Time of Many Worlds* (New York and London: Blackwell, 2004); see also his earlier book for the New Studies in Christian Ethics series, *Responsibility and Christian Ethics* (Cambridge: Cambridge University Press, 1995).

[44] Koenig, *Spirituality in Patient Care*, p. 81.

[45] Sloan, Bagiella and Powell, 'Viewpoint: Religion, Spirituality and Medicine', p. 666. For an earlier British discussion see Kenneth Howe, *Religion, Spirituality and Older People* (Centre for Policy on Ageing, 25–31 Ironmonger Row, London, ECIV 3QP, 1999), chapter 3.

the patients will have once they go back home'.[46] So, for example, it is not just questions about smoking and drinking that are justifiable on this basis, but also about sexual activity and other areas of personal behaviour. So why not Third-Level Faith as well? In addition, he argues:

In fact, all counselling with regard to health maintenance or disease prevention runs the risk of making patients feel guilty if they don't follow recommendations and end up sick. Even recommendations to participate in a support group or social activity can cause guilt in the person who remains reclusive and then develops a recurrence of disease. Does the fear of inducing guilt prevent physicians from addressing these issues or making enquiries? No, it does not. Nor should it stop them from doing a spiritual assessment.[47]

It is at this point that Koenig almost crosses the line into an instrumental understanding of religion: i.e. Third-Level Faith has clear health benefits, so doctors should make a 'spiritual assessment' of their patients with a view to recommending these benefits to them. Koenig does, though, recognise that not all patients will respond to this (in that event the doctor should simply move on), that there may be other secular forms of social support that benefit patients instead, and that both religious and non-religious patients alike will finally die. So, he admits, 'it is impossible and often completely faulty to conclude that a patient's poor physical health is due to lack of faith – and physicians should never even imply this'.[48]

A similar, theologically flawed, instrumentalism may bedevil some of the empirical studies of prayer criticised on methodological grounds by Sloan, Bagiella and Powell. They depict one of the most celebrated as follows:

In this double-blind study, patients in a coronary-care unit were assigned randomly either to standard care or to daily intercessory prayer ministered by three to seven born-again Christians. 29 outcome variables were measured, and on six the prayer group had fewer newly diagnosed ailments. However, the six significant outcomes were not independent: the prayer group had fewer cases of newly diagnosed heart failure and of newly

---

[46] Koenig, *Spirituality in Patient Care*, pp. 83–4.
[47] Koenig, *Spirituality in Patient Care*, pp. 85–6.
[48] Koenig, *Spirituality in Patient Care*, p. 86.

prescribed diuretics and fewer cases of newly diagnosed pneumonia and of newly prescribed antibiotics. There was no control for multiple comparison, a fact recognised by the author.[49]

Now suppose that all of these methodological defects have been overcome (as they may well have been) and that the results for the group receiving the prayers of the born-again Christians were significantly better than those for the control group (using appropriate multivariate models), would that 'prove' that intercessory prayer works? Sceptics would need to be convinced that there was no chicanery or unintended disclosure involved, that the experiment was thoroughly repeatable, that groups of once-born and born-again prayers were properly compared, that Christian prayers were compared with Islamic or Jewish prayers . . . and so on. But, in the end, what would all of these research projects really prove? That prayer can be treated instrumentally? That prayer can be effective when used in a spirit of experimentation rather than prayerfulness? That, if the right prayers are used and the right people are using them, then they can be thoroughly efficacious even if those prayed for actively disbelieve in the power of prayer? All of this is so far removed from an adequately theological understanding of prayer that it is difficult to take it seriously. Even the Synoptic Jesus 'did not do many deeds of power there, because of their unbelief' (Matt. 13.58).

Perhaps the secular significance of health and religion studies is less about trying to prove divine efficaciousness than about challenging a pluralistic age to take worshipping communities more seriously. Within a worshipping community, faith – in the third sense of faith as a response to God – belongs to a continuum within the healing process. While healing is obviously possible without this third level being made explicit, elements of it are likely to be implicit within many healings contexts. It is also at this level that the moral gap between the demand of moral duty and human propensity to selfishness can be narrowed. For the medical professional, especially when grounded in a worshipping community, faith in this third sense offers a powerful source of motivation to act selflessly. For the patient

---

[49] Sloan, Bagiella and Powell, 'Viewpoint: Religion, Spirituality and Medicine', p. 666. The study cited is R. C. Byrd, 'Positive Therapeutic Effects of Intercessory Prayer in a Coronary Care Unit Population', *Southern Medical Journal*, 81 (1988), pp. 826–9.

such a community can also narrow the gap between personal resonance and a shared understanding of cosmic order. Even if an understanding of cosmic order is not shared by both the healer and the one
who is to be healed, it can be explicitly shared by one or the other
party with a worshipping community (especially a community that
has regular intercessions for the ill and needy).

To return to a distinction that I have made elsewhere,[50] public
theology has, I believe, a threefold critical role – criticising, deepening
and widening the ethical debate in society at large. The deepening and
widening aspects depend upon theistic and Christological assumptions, offering a vision for those who will hear of how things could be if
all shared these assumptions and were committed to a Christian
eschaton. Whereas I do not believe that the second and third functions
can play a role in the direct work of public bodies concerned with
ethics, they can and do play a role in the lives of individual patients and
medical professionals. Indeed, as suggested earlier, philosophers such
as Onora O'Neill may underplay the extent to which specifically
religious faith may be important if 'trust' is really to be restored in
the health service today. In the next chapter I will argue that trust also
needs to be accompanied by humility (itself with important theological
roots) in an adequate account of health care ethics.

If health and religion studies are interpreted from this perspective,
then their findings accord more closely with my own findings in
Churchgoing and Christian Ethics. The broad patterns of increased
faith, teleology and altruism found there especially among the most
regular churchgoers (across denominations) do seem to be replicated
in many health and religion studies. So when, as already seen, Koenig
reports that 'of 100 studies in the past century that examined these
relationships, 79 found that religious persons had significantly
greater well-being, life satisfaction, or happiness than did those
who were less religious',[51] he could almost have been referring to
the studies examined in *Churchgoing and Christian Ethics*. In the
latter (as for Koenig) it is not that teleology and altruism are absent
from the general population, it is rather that both are to be found

[50] See Robin Gill, *Moral Leadership in a Postmodern Age* (Edinburgh: T. & T. Clark, 1997),
pp. 6f.
[51] Koenig, *Spirituality in Patient Care*, p. 10.

disproportionately among regular churchgoers. There are also a number of 'mediating structures' to be found among regular church-goers – such as decreased smoking, alcohol consumption and sexual promiscuity and increased social support networks – that incidentally appear to have health benefits too.

For many regular worshippers these health benefits may be both surprising and incidental. Largely unnoticed at the time, they are unlikely to be among the most obvious reasons for them becoming regular worshippers in the first place. And, for many secularists, regular churchgoing may, frankly, be too heavy a price for increased health and longevity. Better to enjoy a shorter and less healthy life than to endure a life-time of religious services that they cannot abide. For neither party does a social policy commending regular worship for its health benefits make much sense.

Yet the empirical connection discovered between regular worship and health does still have some social policy implications, especially about hospital chaplaincy. In Britain, as a result of changes in hospital funding, there has recently been a major review of hospital chaplaincy provision. In a less pluralistic age the statutory provision of Christian hospital chaplains and hospital chapels met compar-atively little opposition. It was also often assumed that hospital chaplains, like other health care professionals, could have ready access to patient notes without patient consent and might even be included in confidential clinical panels. Regular worship (predominantly Anglican in England and Presbyterian in Scotland) was provided in hospital chapels for patients and staff and sometimes on open wards as well. However sceptical individual doctors or nurses might be, hospital chaplaincy was built into and funded by the National Health Service.

In a more pluralistic age today such a pattern of hospital chap-laincy has inevitably been questioned. For a while it also seemed that publicly funded hospital chaplaincy might be discontinued. Some argued (perhaps unaware of health and religion studies) that finite public funds should not be spent on something that lacks clear health benefits. Others argued that, whether or not hospital cha-plains bring health benefits to patients who are religious believers, it is inappropriate that they should be publicly funded or treated as quasi-health-care professionals. Others again maintained that paid hospital chaplains and hospital chapels should more closely represent the religious pluralism of society at large.

To date, state-funded hospital chaplains in Britain have so far survived this review, but they have experienced some radical and continuing changes. There is now a greater emphasis upon 'spirituality' in their work (since 'spirituality is considered to apply both to those who see themselves as 'religious' and to, at least some of, those who do not) and an increased religious pluralism among their number (there are now paid Muslim chaplains in the National Health Service).

Tristram Engelhardt, as noted in passing in chapter 2, sees a radical polarisation emerging from a parallel change in hospital chaplaincy in the United States. For him this change reflects not simply increasing social pluralism, but 'culture wars' in a post-Christian world. He believes that 'traditional Christianity has become discordant with contemporary public sentiments . . . moral and theological sensibilities divide not just Christian from post-Christian and non-Christian, but Christian from Christian, bringing into question the possibility of a unified moral understanding in the once Christian West'.[52] For Engelhardt, the changing role of hospital chaplains offers a clear example of this process (to continue the quote cited earlier):

Once chaplaincy is defined by fully ecumenical professional norms, justifiable with the public discourse of a secular public space, chaplaincy takes on an identity independent of and hostile to traditional Christian concerns. Unlike medicine where Christian physicians may more plausibly address many central professional concerns without reference to their Christian identity (e.g., the diagnosis and treatment of disease may seem the same irrespective of one's religious commitments), chaplaincy is centrally tied to right worship and right belief. Those who do not acknowledge this threat to the authentic Christian identity of chaplains likely hold that the emerging profession of chaplaincy can embrace numerous religious narratives and accounts of spirituality without imposing one of its own. Yet, compassing a plurality of spiritualities in a secular-ecumenical unity threatens to discount the unique truth of the Christian message within a polytheism of religious perspectives . . .[53]

---

[52] H. Tristram Engelhardt Jr, 'The Dechristianization of Christian Hospital Chaplaincy: some Bioethics Reflections on Professionalization, Ecumenization, and Secularization', *Christian Bioethics*, 9:1 (2003), pp. 141–2.

[53] Engelhardt, 'The Dechristianization of Christian Hospital Chaplaincy', p. 140.

Engelhardt characteristically exacerbates 'culture wars' here by using the adjectives 'traditional', 'right', 'authentic' and 'unique' to denote (his understanding of) Christian faith and by caricaturing the emerging concept of chaplaincy (which he dislikes) as 'polytheism'. He then encourages 'choosing sides in the culture wars' in favour of hospital chaplains (among other roles): 'helping patients to step out of immoral relationships such as sexual liaisons outside of the marriage of husband and wife'; 'leading [patients] to wholehearted repentance and conversion in tears and sorrow'; aiding hospital physicians 'refusing to employ medical science in sinful ways (e.g., abortion)'; and 'approving the use of medicine only when it will not distract from the primary goals of repentance and conversion (e.g., recommending to patients that they should refuse treatment which would consume their life in the pursuit of cure and the restoration of health)'; and 'encouraging health care professionals and health care institutions not to participate in interventions forbidden by traditional Christian norms (including refusing to refer to those who would provide such interventions)'.[54]

With such a theological purist remit it is difficult to imagine many state hospitals allowing chaplains any contact at all with their patients. It is unlikely that chaplains who lectured patients on their sexual liaisons, reducing them to 'tears and sorrow', would be regarded as appropriate at their bedsides. Hospital administrators might be concerned about such chaplains contacting medical staff as well. The final parenthesis, for example, would make doctors opposing abortion unemployable in many clinical settings of both hospitals and general practice in the British National Health Service. Even if doctors are strongly opposed to abortion on religious grounds – believing that abortion is indeed murder – they are still required to refer women seeking legally justifiable abortion to other doctors who are not themselves opposed to abortion.

For many decades hospital chaplaincy may only have survived in state hospitals because theological realism has been dominant in its approach to health care ethics. This has allowed hospital chaplains to care compassionately for patients and staff, to respect confidences of both, to minister to the terminally ill, and to comfort the bereaved.

---

[54] Engelhardt, 'The Dechristianization of Christian Hospital Chaplaincy', pp. 145–6.

Those with first-hand experience of hospital chaplaincy will know that in Britain today (when so many people lack formal church connections) it is frequently the hospital chaplain who is asked by families to take the funerals of those who die in hospital. All of this compassionate care would be lost if hospital chaplaincy were abandoned by secular authorities that discerned no connection between health and religion and saw only the fruits of 'culture wars'. Fortunately, religious faith, through state-funded (albeit transformed) hospital chaplaincy, does still have this public function of compassionate care even in pluralistic Britain today.

As has been seen, faith is multi-layered. At a very basic level it involves trust, trust in medical professionals and in the health care that they deliver. However, at a deeper level it involves profound beliefs, commitments and values. Even in a pluralistic and supposedly 'secular' society, it would be surprising if it did not also involve religious orientations and convictions. Without over-stating the evidence from the increasing number of empirical studies suggesting that there is an important connection between health/well-being and religious belief and belonging, it does seem that faith at all levels is relevant to health care even within a pluralistic society. For the Synoptic Jesus it was crucial to healing and wholeness. Perhaps, after all, it still is today.

CHAPTER 7

Humility in health care ethics

Finally there is humility within health care ethics. In a context of exaggerated claims made in the name of medical (especially genetic) science and seemingly unlimited patient demand, this fourth virtue is particularly apposite today. Within medicine humility in a moral sense is to be distinguished from etiquette. In terms of etiquette it is good manners not to boast about being able to do something even when there are grounds for believing that it can be done. However, as a moral term, humility involves a proper recognition both of personal frailty (and, thus, of the need for personal temperance and restraint) and of the role of others in achieving something. For the medical professional there is a constant temptation to claim too much authority and knowledge (a temptation in which patients themselves frequently conspire). Regrettably, there is also a parallel temptation for theologians engaged in health care ethics to claim too much (divine) authority and (revealed) knowledge.

An emphasis upon reticence, temperance or humility is certainly not unique to Christianity. Confucianism advises leaders to retain the respect of their people and Buddhism, in at least some of its forms, encourages detachment from excessive and unrealistic desires: both have been powerful carriers of humility. Within theistic traditions there is a particular reason for the importance of temperance and humility. The Qu'ran, like the Jewish and Christian scriptures, expresses this frequently: given their belief in God as creator, human beings as creatures should indeed be humble, temperate and restrained. So, having commanded them to give alms to the needy, the faithful are immediately reminded:

God is He that created you, then He provided for you, then He shall make you dead, and then He shall give you life; is there any of your associates does aught of that? Glory be to Him! High be He exalted above that they associate![1]

In chapter 3 a pattern of Jesus' reticence in a context of exaggerated crowd expectations was detected within and surrounding the Synoptic healing stories. At the conclusion of several stories Jesus commands that no one should be told: in the instruction to the demons (Mark 1.34 / Luke 4.41); to the leper (Mark 1.44 / Matt. 8.4 / Luke 5.14); to the unclean spirits (Mark 3.12 / Matt. 12.16); to Jairus' family (Mark 5.43 / Luke 8.56); to the deaf-mute (Mark 7.36); and to the two blind men (Matt. 9.30). In addition the blind man is told 'Do not even enter the village' after his healing (Mark 8.26). Clearly this feature is most common in Mark. Crowd amazement/fear also occurs frequently at the end of a number of stories in Mark: the man in the synagogue (1.27), the paralytic (2.12), the Gadarene demoniac (5.15), Jairus' daughter (5.42) and the deaf-mute (7.37). Although Matthew omits four of these commands to silence while adding only one (leading to the speculation that Mark alone is committed to the so-called 'messianic secret'), I argued that a careful analysis of the sequence of events in Matthew 8–9 shows a very similar overall pattern of reticence, movement and troubled crowds with Jesus commanding the leper to silence (8.4), being troubled by crowds (8.18), trying to escape (8.28), but crowds returning (8.34) and so on.

But what of Luke? After all it is Luke who recounts three occasions when this reticence was apparently abandoned: the instruction to John the Baptist's disciples to 'Go and tell John what you have seen and heard: the blind receive their sight, the lame walk, the lepers are cleansed, the deaf hear, the dead are raised' (Luke 7.22 / Matt. 11.4–5); the instruction to the Gadarene demoniac to go home and tell what 'the Lord' (in Mark) or 'God' (in Luke) 'has done for you' (Mark 5.19 / Luke 8.39); and the instruction to the Pharisees to tell Herod, 'Go tell that old fox for me, "Listen, I am casting out demons and performing cures today and tomorrow"' (Luke 13.32).

Here, too, context is important. That third caustic instruction, unique to Luke, hardly appears as a boast. It is preceded by the

---

[1] Sura xxx.39. The translation of the Qu'ran used is Arthur J. Arberry, *The Koran Interpreted* (Oxford: Oxford University Press, 1998).

contentious healing on the Sabbath of a woman crippled for eighteen years (13.10–17) in which Jesus denounces the leader of the synagogue and the surrounding crowd as 'You hypocrites' (13.15). And it is followed immediately by Jesus acknowledging that 'I must be on my way, because it is impossible for a prophet to be killed outside Jerusalem' (13.33) and his lament over Jerusalem. This, in turn, is followed by another contentious healing on the Sabbath (14.1–6) and by the parable about humility (14.7–14).

The first instruction, unique to the common source of Matthew and Luke, does seem more akin to a boast. In Luke it is also preceded by two non-contentious healing stories, the healing of the centurion's servant (7.1–10) and the raising of the widow's son at Nain (7.11–17). In the first story Jesus is amazed and tells the crowd, 'I tell you, not even in Israel have I found such faith' (7.9) and in the second it is the crowd who, seized with fear, say, 'A great prophet has risen among us!' (7.16). Yet both Luke and Matthew conclude this 'boast' with a self-deprecating, ironic comparison by Jesus: 'For John the Baptist has come eating no bread and drinking no wine, and you say, "He has a demon"; the Son of Man has come eating and drinking, and you say, "Look, a glutton and a drunkard, a friend of tax collectors and sinners!"' (Luke 7.33–4 / Matt. 11.18–19).

However, it is the way that Luke changes and embellishes material which he has otherwise copied that is probably most revealing. These alterations suggest that Luke does indeed share with Mark and Matthew a similar pattern of reticence in a context of exaggerated crowd expectations within and surrounding the healing stories. For example, Luke copies from Mark the commands to tell no one given both to the demons (Mark 1.34 / Luke 4.41) and to the leper (Mark 1.44 / Luke 5.14). Yet, immediately after the first of these, when Jesus went away to pray in a deserted place, instead of following Mark's account of Simon and his companions hunting for him and saying 'Everyone is searching for you', Luke much more explicitly writes: 'And the crowds were looking for him; and when they reached him, they wanted to prevent him from leaving them' (4.42). He then gives the account of the calling of the first disciples and the draught of fish, mentioning at the outset that 'the crowd was pressing in on him' (5.1). The crowd reappears after the cleansing of the leper and then Luke adds: 'But he would withdraw to deserted places and pray' (5.16).

In the following story, the healing of the paralytic, Luke copies Mark's conclusion about the crowd amazement, but embellishes it adding that they 'were filled with awe', saying 'We have seen strange things [*paradoxa*] today' (5.26). In the next chapter Luke again embellishes Mark's story, this time that of the healing of the man with the withered hand by adding that the Pharisees 'were filled with fury' (6.11). At every point Jesus' reticence is strongly associated with exaggerated crowd expectations and even with crowd hostility.

In all three Synoptic Gospels, despite some variations, there is a common pattern of reticence/humility in relation to healing. Particularly troublesome to the Synoptic Jesus are those who deliberately disobey his command to silence. Matthew's story of the healing of the two blind men captures this exactly: 'And their eyes were opened. Then Jesus sternly ordered them, "See that no one knows of this." But they went away and spread the news about him throughout that district' (9.30–1). It was seen earlier that, although explicit commands to silence are absent from the healing stories in the Fourth Gospel and Acts, there is evidence even in them of exaggerated and troublesome crowd expectations surrounding these acts of healing. Of course it is within a context of such crowd expectations that the boastful claims of ancient or modern faith healers become so damaging.

This pattern contrasts sharply with reports of some Pentecostal healing missions today. Morris Cerullo's Mission to London in the early 1990s again provides an instructive example. In her sociological account of this Nancy Schaefer shows how Cerullo first set up his own independent ministry in 1961, working from his garage in San Diego. He established a monthly magazine, *Deeper Life*, and within five years was holding conferences to attract recent charismatic converts. Ten years later he began to produce television programmes, eventually entitled *Victory with Morris Cerullo*. In 1990 he acquired Global Satellite Network (formerly owned by the now disgraced evangelist Jim Bakker). By 1992 his publishing and broadcasting network was valued at £27,000,000 and he was holding evangelistic crusades in more than seventy countries, with a stated ambition to 'win a billion souls' by 2000.

During the summer of 1992 Cerullo's Mission to London launched an advertising campaign with billboards placed at various strategic points around London and publicity given out in many local evangelical and Pentecostal churches. Posters featured discarded white canes and overturned wheelchairs and carried the caption 'Some Will See Miracles For the First Time'. By October 'after investigating complaints, the Advertising Standards Authority found that the posters had "targeted on the disabled" and were a source of distress'.[2]

Schaefer describes in detail a typical day at Cerullo's Mission to London in August 1994. It lasted from 10am to 10pm and apparently attracted a predominantly Afro-Caribbean following. The start of the day consisted of a variety of booths in the exhibition hall selling Christian books, videos, t-shirts and bumper-stickers, among other similar items. At 11.30am there was a service, made up of singing and intercessory prayers, 'followed by personal testimonials of miraculous healing given by a different individual each day'. Then followed four consecutive hour-long teaching sessions 'which covered topics ranging from eschatology and adventism to generational curses and spiritual warfare'.[3] The healing service itself, open to a wider public, was then held in the evening. At this Cerullo played the central role, talking 'in a folksy vernacular . . . main points are repeated in easy-to-remember phrases ("The Devil is a liar") and are illustrated in stories rather than defended through complex theological argument':[4]

As the service progresses, the milieu begins to change perceptively. At first the American speaks slowly in a quiet voice but gradually increases the tempo and volume of his delivery, until he virtually shouts at the top of his voice in rapid successive bursts. The crowd roars its approval on cues given by him and they respond enthusiastically with shouts of 'Amen' and 'Thank you Jesus'. At times the cacophony in the hall is almost deafening as some exuberant attendees become 'slain in the Spirit'. They shout, laugh, weep, dance, wave, clap, collapse, speak in tongues and cast out demonic spirits . . . Meanwhile Cerullo describes the outpouring of the Holy Spirit as 'liquid fire' and calls out ailments which purportedly are being healed . . . He

---

[2] Nancy A. Schaefer, 'Making the Rulers Tremble!: Morris Cerullo World Evangelism's 1994 Mission to London Revival', in Marion Bowman (ed.), *Healing and Religion* (Enfield Lock, Middlesex: Hisarlik Press, 2000), p. 29.
[3] Schaefer, 'Making the Rulers Tremble', p. 25.
[4] Schaefer, 'Making the Rulers Tremble', p. 27.

then proceeds to give out the invitation to come forward (the altar call) and asks those who have been healed to come on the stage. Individuals then give their personal testimonials in turn; Cerullo prays and lays hands over each one. Ordinarily people collapse when touched and volunteers stand by to catch them as they fall. This portion of the service can be quite lengthy depending upon the number of people who come forward ... Cerullo usually allows anywhere [between] twelve or more testimonials before concluding the service. A closing hymn is then sung but one which is quiet and calming rather than loud and rousing as sung at the outset.[5]

The difference between this and the Synoptic Gospels' reticence is striking. For Cerullo maximum publicity, sensational advertising, animated crowds and a carefully orchestrated healing service were crucial. There was no command from him to tell no one. There was no putting distraught relatives out of the room while the vulnerable were healed in private. Instead healing was set on a public stage in a large hall and with excited friends and relatives singing, dancing and shouting. And, of course, there was no attempt by Cerullo to escape from the pressing crowds and exaggerated claims to find a place of solitude for prayer. The crowds did not need to go hunting for Cerullo, he was already seeking them. Moreover, there were considerable amounts of money involved and an extensive commercial empire. Cerullo, an exponent of the so-called 'Gospel of Prosperity', was a forerunner of what Jeremy Carrette and Philip King now identify as a growing phenomenon in a pluralistic society of commercialised 'selling spirituality'.[6] In short, the reticence and humility of the Synoptic Jesus in the context of healing was replaced with vociferous and systematic boasts of one claiming that 'Some Will See Miracles For the First Time'.

An important connection between compassionate care and humility emerges from this example. In the absence of humility many people are harmed. As mentioned in the previous chapter, apparently a woman died after attending Morris Cerullo's 1992 Mission to London as a result of stopping her medication. Disabled groups felt that they had been 'targeted' and distressed by the aggressive advertising. Members of the over-excited crowd may have felt seriously

---

[5] Schaefer, 'Making the Rulers Tremble', pp. 27–8.
[6] Jeremy Carrette and Philip King, *Selling Spirituality?* (London: Routledge, 2005).

duped and swindled once they reflected in tranquillity afterwards. Those on the fringes of churches may have experienced profound disillusionment about Christian faith as a result of experiencing this mission. In contrast, the Synoptic Jesus' reticence may have been important in preventing effervescent crowds from inflicting self-harm and, indeed, harm to others in their attempt 'to prevent him from leaving them' (Luke 4.42).

Jean Porter's *Moral Action and Christian Ethics*, within the New Studies in Christian Ethics series, offers a valuable account of how the Christian virtues of compassionate care and humility connect. In her reformulation of Aquinas' account of the interrelationship of virtues she distinguishes between the cardinal, self-regarding virtues, such as temperance and fortitude, and other-regarding virtues, such as kindness, compassion and care. The self-regarding virtues are considered, by both Porter and Aquinas, as essential if a moral agent is to act at all. So, if temperance is seen today as self-control or self-restraint, then, if individuals are wholly unable to control or restrain themselves, they will also be incapable of acting as self-determining moral agents. Some degree of self-control or self-restraint is a prerequisite of moral action:

an agent who did not possess these qualities at all would be able to perform discrete actions, but she would not be able to do most of the things that involve sustaining a course of activity; the fulfilment of role responsibilities, the pursuit of aims that can only be attained by a series of actions, participation in most social actions, promising, contracting, all these would be prohibitively difficult for her.[7]

Other-regarding virtues are also important if individuals are to be persuaded to consider the needs of other people beyond themselves, although it is not always obvious how these virtues relate to self-regarding virtues. For example, if the other-regarding virtue of justice is considered, 'a just person may well do something unjust, and, conversely, an unjust person may act justly, and yet in each case what is relevant to evaluating the particular action (*qua* act of justice) is simply its conformity to norms of equity and non-maleficence ...

[7] Jean Porter, *Moral Action and Christian Ethics* (Cambridge: Cambridge University Press, 1995), pp. 171–2.

the acts of justice appear to have little or no organic connection with the agent's character'.[8] Porter acknowledges that the so-called psychopath 'combines a capacity for manipulation with murderous indifference to human life', yet:

None the less ... the psychopath needs some capacities for empathy for others to function as a human person at all. Just as the individual who is altogether deprived of the capacities for self-restraint and courage crosses the line from vice (or addiction) to outright insanity, so the person who has no capacities at all for fellow-feeling will be incapable of any but the most rudimentary kinds of actions. Thus, while it is not necessary to possess the *virtues* of concern for others, sympathy, kindness, and the like in order to function as an agent, none the less, this family of virtues draws upon, and perfects, qualities which are essential to the functioning of the agent, *qua* agent. It would be reasonable to assume that these sorts of virtues are desirable, are, in a broad sense, beneficial to the agent herself, as well as to those around her.[9]

Now, of course, the determinedly callous, manipulative or selfish person is unlikely to be convinced by this. However, Porter is convinced that most people 'do retain some desire for a dignified human life, which includes some openness to learning and aesthetic experience for their own sakes, and, similarly, most people do care, at least a little, about some other persons, and want to be open to the presence of others in their lives'. So, for them at least, 'the virtues of care for others are internally connected in some ways to the good of the agent herself, as well as being of benefit to others'.[10]

In that sense, self-regarding virtues (e.g. reticence and humility) are connected within the lives of most people to other-regarding virtues (e.g. compassion and care). In a healing context, reticence/humility is an important perquisite of compassionate care, and compassionate care reinforces this reticence/humility. Conversely, the boastful, self-seeking healer considerably endangers the compassionate care of others (in order to gain their esteem or money or both) and that, in turn, shapes a healer who (despite pretensions to the contrary) is actually more callous than compassionate or caring. Perhaps it is just that that leads Jesus in Luke to the rebuke

---

[8] Porter, *Moral Action*, p. 180.   [9] Porter, *Moral Action*, p. 184.
[10] Porter, *Moral Action*, p. 185.

(characteristically applied in the Synoptic Gospels to those in positions of religious responsibility) 'You hypocrites' (13.15). Hypocrites here take on the meaning, not simply of actors who wear masks, but of those religious people who claim to be acting in principled ways but are actually failing to show compassionate care to those in serious need.

Just as the Synoptic healing stories seem to connect other-regarding and self-regarding virtues, so it appears does Paul. Both sets of virtues are placed together in Galatians:

The fruit of the Spirit is love, joy, peace, patience, kindness, generosity, faithfulness, gentleness, and self-control. There is no law against such things. And those who belong to Christ Jesus have crucified the flesh with its passions and desires. If we live by the Spirit, let us also be guided by the Spirit. Let us not become conceited, competing against one another, envying one another. (Gal. 5.22–6)

Kindness and generosity (and, negatively, competition and envy) are clearly other-regarding, and gentleness and self-control (and, negatively, conceit) are self-regarding: love, faithfulness, joy, peace and patience could be either or both. As Porter observes, 'if it is true that the virtues of caring are internally connected to the good of the agent herself, one consequence is that we cannot draw a sharp distinction between self-regarding and other-regarding virtues'.[11] Humility and compassionate care, especially in an effective and ethical context of healing, flow backwards and forwards into each other.

As do humility and faith. Faith in God – for Jews, Christians and Muslims alike – is often given as a central reason for humility. Worshippers in each of these traditions know that it is not they who should be worshipped by others but God alone who is to be worshipped. And humility may be important in healers if others are to trust/have faith in them.

David H. Smith provides an important illustration of this when discussing the relationship between nurses and doctors in caring for the dying. As part of a wider project of the role of religion in the life of professionals involved in this caring, Smith interviewed ten Christian nurses with mixed experience of oncology wards and hospices in the

---

[11] Porter, *Moral Action*, p. 186.

United States. They were all female and of mixed ages and denominations. Some were evangelicals, three were Catholics, and most of the others went to Methodist or Presbyterian churches with varying degrees of regularity. All 'take comfort in their religious beliefs', yet 'most of them offer trenchant criticisms of religion and its presence or absence in the clinical setting'.[12] Smith found it 'striking that religious institutions or clergy are seldom looked to for either comfort or teaching, either by evangelicals or the mainline professionals ... respondents are unlikely to turn to clergy when they need someone to talk to'. For many of these respondents, 'the way religion might help is not ideological or dogmatic; rather it sustains another dimension of life, one that serves both to change the subject and provide a broader and richer perspective through which tragedies at the end of life can be reenvisioned, or put into another perspective'.[13]

In his article Smith views the role of nurses in a clinical setting of caring for the dying basically from their perspective. He is particularly interested in the occasions when this role involves nurses in tension or even conflict with others. He reports that his respondents are very aware that nurses and doctors often have very different expectations: 'no one will fault a nurse for the fact that someone dies under her care – so long as the technical assignment has been handled properly – but they will certainly fault a physician for an unanticipated death'.[14] This can and does lead to conflict:

Everyone who has been a nurse, talked to a nurse, or read about nursing knows that conflicts with physicians are a significant part of a nurse's agenda. One dimension of this conflict concerns quality control in medical care. Nurses have an increasingly high level of scientific and technical preparation and competence, and they think this technical competence is the sine qua non of their professional work. They may find themselves able to correct a physician's orders and prevent mistakes. For example, we were told of an incident in which a physician had written an incorrect prescription. When a nurse caught the mistake, the physician's first response was a raw exercise of authority: 'Do it!' But the nurse persevered and involved her

---

[12] David H. Smith, 'Professional Commitment to Personal Care: Nurses' Commitments in Care for the Dying', in David H. Smith (ed.), *Caring Well: Religion, Narrative, and Health Care Ethics* (Louisville, KY: Westminster John Knox Press, 2000), p. 223.
[13] Smith, 'Professional Commitment to Personal Care', p. 224.
[14] Smith, 'Professional Commitment to Personal Care', p. 229.

superior, who raised the issue again offstage with the physician. At last the physician admitted her mistake and apologized.[15]

This clash of authority is highly instructive. Smith singles out the 'importance of courage and diplomatic skills in a nurse's set of virtues ... without courage, the nurse would not have pointed out the mistake, and the patient might have been harmed or even killed ... without diplomatic skills, conflict with physicians would lead to acrimonious standoffs'.[16] But there were also some virtues that were needed by the doctor in this story. It can doubtless be very difficult to be humble in a clinical setting where roles are differentiated and then publicly challenged. An authoritarian command, without properly looking at whether the challenge is justified, is very tempting. Yet it might also be very damaging to the patient. The patient does need to trust/have faith in both the doctor and the nurse, and the nurse and the doctor will work better together if they in turn trust/have faith in each other. However, humility is also needed if each of these parties is to avoid arrogance and the mistakes that can come with arrogance.

Perhaps it is this humility that is one of the crucial ingredients too underplayed in Onora O'Neill's analysis examined in the previous chapter. She puzzles about why in Western society 'public trust in medicine, science and biotechnology has seemingly faltered'.[17] And she finally places much of the blame on the audit agenda and the openness agenda that have been so extensively deployed over the last twenty years in order to improve accountability, and with it trustworthiness, in many areas of public life. It is possible, however, that at least part of the blame may lie at the feet of exponents of medicine, science and technology for making exaggerated claims.

In the areas of biotechnology and gene therapy, in particular, there has been much excitement, hyperbole and public fear. Articles and programmes in the media have simultaneously raised high public expectations and generated considerable public suspicion. Theologians, too, as was seen in chapter 2, have sometimes played a

---

[15] Smith, 'Professional Commitment to Personal Care', p. 227.

[16] Smith, 'Professional Commitment to Personal Care', p. 227.

[17] Onora O'Neill, *Autonomy and Trust in Bioethics* (Cambridge: Cambridge University Press, 2002), p. 3.

public role in generating this suspicion. Having been involved with British regulatory bodies in gene therapy and embryonic stem cell research over the last decade, I have become thoroughly acquainted with exaggerated claims both from members of the scientific community and from fellow theologians. In February 1993 permission was given in Britain for the first gene-transfer experiment – an attempt to benefit children with adenosine deaminase (ADA) deficiency. There was considerable optimism at this stage that gene therapy would soon be able to deliver therapeutic benefit to patients with malignant tumours, cystic fibrosis, and many other inherited disorders caused by single defective genes. A dozen years later this optimism has been considerably tempered, as Celia Deane-Drumond's recent *Genetics and Christian Ethics*[18] shows clearly in the New Studies in Christian Ethics series. It has proved very much more difficult than some thought at the time to find effective and safe ways of transferring genes. Not only does the body resist such transfers, but, even when ways are discovered to circumvent resistance, it has proved extremely difficult to target gene transfers without causing serious risks to the patient (such as leukaemia) or, more worryingly, to any future offspring (as a result of affecting the patient's semen or ova).[19] Consequently, an area of very considerable excitement in medical science has now become much more reticent. It is possible that the current optimism surrounding stem cell research (given high-profile publicity by the courageous actor Christopher Reeve) may encounter similar set-backs and disappointments. Those theologians (such as myself) who have cautiously supported such research would be wise to be alert to this. Nonetheless, such caution is not to be confused with the theological hyperbole criticised in chapter 2. I believe that Audrey Chapman, like Deane-Drumond, is right to criticise theologians who claim too readily that scientists working in these novel areas are now 'playing God'.[20] Similarly Derek Burke is right to condemn exaggerated

---

[18] Celia Deane-Drumond, *Genetics and Christian Ethics* (Cambridge: Cambridge University Press, 2005).
[19] See Jonathan Kimmelman, 'Recent Developments in Gene Transfer: Risk and Ethics', *British Medical Journal*, 330:53 (8 January 2005), pp. 79–82.
[20] See Audrey R. Chapman, *Unprecedented Choices: Religious Ethics at the Frontiers of Genetic Science* (Minneapolis: Fortress Press, 1999), chapter 3.

theological claims in his own specialist area of the genetic modification of food.[21] A balance of cautious trust and humility is needed by both scientists and theologians here.

Darlene Fozard Weaver's *Self Love and Christian Ethics*, also in the New Studies in Christian Ethics series, offers a different way of balancing self-regarding and other-regarding virtues. She argues that an adequate Christian concept of 'love' or *agape* should be both self-regarding and other-regarding, and that these two aspects of love are interdependent. Like many of the other Christian and secular ethicists already reviewed – such as Chapman and O'Neill – Weaver is unimpressed by individualistic understandings of autonomy that dominate some accounts of health care ethics. From her perspective of seeking to defend self-love, she argues that these are often based upon what she terms 'the norm of self-realization': 'this norm refers to the dominant subjectivism of recent work in ethics in particular and contemporary culture in general, a shift towards voluntaristic and intuitionistic understandings of the moral good, in which moral values are primarily matters of personal or communal choice and moral obligations are taken to be largely situation-specific'.[22] The claim of the secular bioethicist John Harris (cited in the previous chapter) that 'it is only by the exercise of autonomy that our lives become in any sense our own . . . by shaping our lives for ourselves we assert our own values and our individuality',[23] is a very clear example of such a 'norm of self-realization'. Shaping *our* lives for *ourselves* and asserting *our* values and *our* individuality appear to be crucial to Harris. Weaver (following Charles Taylor) would surely argue that this in effect defines autonomy in terms of negative freedom, that is freedom as the absence of constraints:

This negative freedom belongs to a complex of values like self-sufficiency, independence and self-determination. In other words, in autonomy, negative freedom meets the power of self-definition. The tension inherent to this union spawns a confusing mentality in which the power to define and

---

[21] See Derek Burke, 'Genetic Engineering of Food', in Fraser Watts (ed.), *Christians and Bioethics* (London: SPCK, 2000), pp. 21–34.

[22] Darlene Fozard Weaver, *Self Love and Christian Ethics* (Cambridge: Cambridge University Press, 2002), p. 2.

[23] John Harris, 'Consent and End of Life Decisions', *Journal of Medical Ethics*, 29:1 (2003), pp. 10–11.

determine oneself through one's choices and pursuits requires a ... freedom from those very 'commitments' ... To borrow from the world of professional sports, the self is a 'free agent', loosely and provisionally tied to a team, ready and willing to affiliate itself with another one should the terms be – and remain – to its liking.[24]

Such an understanding, Weaver argues, is deeply problematic. It faces difficulties accounting 'for the ways prejudice, habit, convention, and experience can limit freedom even in the absence of external constraints'. It produces a sense of entitlement 'stoked by capitalism', it 'insulates the autonomous self from duty to others and from critic- ism', and it 'threatens to collapse authority into authoritarianism'.[25]

Onora O'Neill might agree with much of this from her Kantian position. Where Weaver differs is in her espousal of a specifically Christian understanding of self-love:

A Christian ethics of self love resists the reduction and distortion of freedom so characteristic of our contemporary Western outlook. When we recognize that the freedom for self-determination is only one aspect of the freedom of and for self-relation we begin to see that we can only know the depth and range of freedom, its power and meaning, its promise and frailty in relation to a source of value that establishes freedom and a real good that beckons it. Put theologically, we know the meaning of freedom in relation to God. Reckoning with our own status as creatures of a God who has in Jesus Christ revealed the divine self as one who acts on our behalf shows the limitations and illusions of autonomy. Freedom is not a capacity for self-definition but for self-disposal or self-commitment.[26]

Weaver follows a long line of theologians from Augustine onwards who see self-love, neighbour-love and God-love as the three inter- dependent features of the dominical commands.

Once the virtue of humility is set into this threefold context it does assume a profounder shape for Christians (and Jews and Muslims). Within almost every act of worship individuals are encouraged to confess their sins, repent and recognise their status as frail creatures. They are then encouraged to thank, glorify and worship God, the Creator and the source of all that is. Finally they are encouraged to go

[24] Weaver, *Self Love and Christian Ethics*, p. 20.
[25] Weaver, *Self Love and Christian Ethics*, p. 20.
[26] Weaver, *Self Love and Christian Ethics*, p. 21.

out into the world to serve and care for other people. The three fundamental liturgical movements of repentance, worship and renewal are ubiquitous accompaniments of the religiously active – reinforcing, in turn, humility, faith and compassionate care – and have few adequate counterparts in modern, secular life.

Another author in New Studies in Christian Ethics who highlights the importance of faith, humility and care in a secular context is Christopher Cook in his *Alcohol, Addiction and Christian Ethics.*[27] His own clinical work in the area of alcohol dependence has convinced him that there is a gap in much secular discussion. While he is critical of simplistic moralistic approaches to alcoholism (especially the nineteenth-century Christian temperance movement) and is deeply informed by modern biosocial studies, he argues that a careful use of Paul and Augustine's notion of the divided self can still make a significant contribution today. The latter can suggest an important link between our experience of ourselves and that of those with a medical disorder of severe alcohol dependence. A proper sense of humility can help us to see that some experience of addiction – whether it involves alcohol, food, sex, or simply shopping – is an everyday reality in which each of us experiences a divided self. In addition, he argues that the need for grace is an essential component in any adequate response to addictive disorders – whether it is the explicit Christian concept of God's grace in Jesus Christ or the rather vaguer notion of the need for 'Higher Power' of Alcoholics Anonymous. Indeed, at an empirical level, he suggests that spiritual or religious experience is often and unsurprisingly associated with recovery from addiction (tortuous as it often is).

HEALTH CARE RATIONING

One of the most intractable areas in modern health care ethics – variously depicted (with different ethical emphasise) as health care rationing, prioritising in health, or allocating scarce medical resources – can be used to understand better the importance of humility in relation to faith and compassionate care. It is not that

---

[27] Christopher Cook, *Alcohol, Addiction and Christian Ethics* (Cambridge: Cambridge University Press, 2006).

humility, on its own, can possibly resolve all of the ethical dilemmas raised by health care rationing in modern, pluralistic societies. Yet humility – understood here as medical professionals not claiming too much and patients not demanding too much – does have an important, but often neglected role to play. Given a human tendency to self-serving arrogance, on the one hand, and to selfishness, on the other, the Synoptic Jesus' humility in the context of healing might still be able to make a significant contribution to health care ethics today in the public forum of a Western, pluralistic society.

Two recent books provide powerful, but contrasting, contributions by Christians to the ethical debate about health care rationing. The first of these is John Butler's *The Ethics of Health Care Rationing*.[28] Butler, a professor of health care studies and also a lay preacher in the Methodist Church, notes briefly that 'the ethics of the New Testament, even though yielding up no particular rules for choosing between competing patients, would place a dominant moral emphasis on the care of those at the bottom of the social pile'. However, he adds immediately that religiously derived values 'are absolute only for those who recognize them as such, and they cannot easily be applied in modern situations of immense complexity that are light-years removed from the cultures in which they originated'.[29] From then onwards he seldom returns to such values. The second book is Tristram Engelhardt and Mark Cherry's collection *Allocating Scarce Medical Resources: Roman Catholic Perspectives*.[30] This book arises from a series of meetings of mostly Roman Catholic theologians and medical doctors attempting to establish what if anything Catholic teaching and theology have to contribute to how scarce medical resources should be allocated. A good deal of the discussion focuses specifically upon intensive care units, noting that these extremely expensive and highly staffed units were originally intended to be temporary mechanisms to allow treatment and restoration of the seriously ill but all too often have become a means of extending the lives of those who are terminally ill. Contributors

---

[28] John Butler, *The Ethics of Health Care Rationing: Principles and Practices* (London: Cassell, 1999).
[29] Butler, *The Ethics of Health Care Rationing*, p. 63.
[30] H. Tristram Engelhardt Jr and Mark J. Cherry (eds.), *Allocating Scarce Medical Resources: Roman Catholic Perspectives* (Washington, DC: Georgetown University Press, 2002).

explore what theology has to say about this shift of function in many modern hospitals, especially in the context of private treatment and (particularly in the US) of over-treatment of the wealthy. In contrast to Butler it is theological throughout. Nevertheless, the various essays in *Allocating Scarce Medical Resources* soon demonstrate that, even when Catholic theologians can agree to use specifically Catholic health care doctrines and distinctions, they find it difficult to resolve their differences about how important they are, how they should be understood, or how they should be applied.

Using British evidence from the 1990s, Butler argues that there is an obvious gap between supply and demand in health care. For example: within renal replacement therapy and intensive cancer therapy there is 'a substantial and sustained shortfall'; older patients have been denied intensive care; alcoholics 'have been turned away' from liver transplantation programmes; effective chemotherapy for ovarian cancer 'is being rationed by health authorities'; rates of coronary bypass surgery 'are lower in Britain than in many other developed countries'; 'fewer than three per cent of couples who might benefit from assisted conception' are receiving treatment; and health authorities 'are quietly dropping certain services from the menu of those they can afford to provide through the NHS'.[31] Many of these shortfalls result from a lack of financial and/or personnel resources, but, in the case of kidney and heart transplants, it is a shortage of donated organs that is the central problem. Details will inevitably fluctuate from one decade to another (such as levels of assisted conception provided under the NHS). However, it is likely that for the foreseeable future every decade will continue to provide similar evidence of a substantial gap between supply and demand in health care in Britain.

Butler then explores a variety of ways that this gap has been or might be reduced. Some of these depend upon explicit rationing ('rationing mechanisms that depend on rules of entitlement') and others upon implicit rationing ('those that depend on the discretion of gatekeepers').[32] Publicly financed health authorities might, for

[31] Butler, *The Ethics of Health Care Rationing*, pp. 8–9.
[32] Butler, *The Ethics of Health Care Rationing*, p. 13.

example, articulate explicit priorities for health care (as Oregon attempted to do after canvassing the electorate's views about priorities), or they might expect hospital consultants to act as gatekeepers deciding which patients should have the most treatment (as happens frequently in the NHS). There are a number of strategies they can adopt: removing services from the menu of those on offer (such as not providing novel forms of IVF on the NHS); relying upon the courts to decide upon difficult cases and to provide 'some initiative for determining rules or rights of access to health services in situations where they are in scarce supply';[33] or reducing patient demand either 'by discouraging patients [sometimes through their GPs or their receptionists] from entering the health care system in the first place (primary inhibitors)' or 'by introducing obstacles that hamper their progress through it [such as waiting lists] once they have got in (secondary inhibitors)'.[34] More positively, the gap might be narrowed through enhancing the efficiency and effectiveness of health care or through refocusing attention towards prevention. Yet, whatever strategies are adopted (and however ethical or unethical they are deemed to be) the 'seemingly intractable imbalance between the demand for, and supply of, health care in publicly funded systems'[35] is likely to remain.

Butler looks at length at the theories of the philosophers John Rawls, Norman Daniels and Len Doyal about the just distribution of resources. For example, Doyal[36] suggests a complex system of priorities: highest priority should be given to ensuring that a fair distribution of care is made within, rather than between, different categories of treatment (for example, it is wrong to give all treatment resources to children and none to the elderly); next, within categories of treatment, priority should be given to patients with the greatest threat that their illness or disability poses to their human 'flourishing'; beyond this, if priorities are still needed, they should be made, not according to the predilection of health care professionals, but randomly; finally,

---

[33] Butler, *The Ethics of Health Care Rationing*, p. 24.
[34] Butler, *The Ethics of Health Care Rationing*, p. 27.
[35] Butler, *The Ethics of Health Care Rationing*, p. 37.
[36] See Len Doyal, 'Needs, Rights and Equity: Moral Quality in Healthcare Rationing', *Quality in Health Care*, 4 (1995), pp. 273–83, and 'The Role of the Public in Health Care Rationing', *Critical Public Health*, 4 (1993), pp. 49–52.

priorities should take into account both effectiveness and the views of the public, should not take into account patients' life-styles, and should be debated openly. However, Butler concludes that such theories do not actually work in the context of the NHS:

The arguments of Rawls, Daniels and Doyal about the just distribution of resources have implications for health care at an institutional level: their insights are to be applied, to the extent that they can be, through the ways in which health care services are structured and organized. Yet ... these notions of distributive justice are expounded at a sufficiently high level of generality to make their translation from drawing board to building site a difficult one. To expect a country's health care system to conform to the architectural requirements articulated by, for example, Doyal, is to assume a degree of political and managerial control over the system, and a level of rational capacity within it, that might be seen, quite simply, as wishful thinking.[37]

Eventually Butler turns away from such theoretical positions, believing that 'no agreed or unambiguous answers are likely to emerge'.[38] He listens, instead, to those actually working within the NHS, using his own discipline of social science rather than moral philosophy. As a result he records thirteen qualitative interviews about rationing with those working on the clinical or administrative sides of the NHS. From these he finds that an awareness of the gap between supply and demand is ubiquitous: 'the language may differ but the sentiment is the same: all informants felt pressured by the lack of resources of one kind or another, and all were having to make a continuous stream of decisions about priorities in their work'.[39] So, the health visitor found her workload excessive, the district nurse reported that rationing ran throughout her work, the GP noted that he now thought in terms of opportunity costs, the psychiatrist found that he was always too busy, and the nurse manager was worried about excessive demands for scarce resources. Such pressure, Butler concludes, 'is an ever-present feature of the health service rather than a transient phenomenon induced by time-limited events which will eventually pass'.[40]

---

[37] Butler, *The Ethics of Health Care Rationing*, p. 96.
[38] Butler, *The Ethics of Health Care Rationing*, p. 234.
[39] Butler, *The Ethics of Health Care Rationing*, p. 221.
[40] Butler, *The Ethics of Health Care Rationing*, p. 221.

Naturally this tended to cause considerable stress among the health care professionals interviewed. It also, so Butler notes, had some undesirable effects upon patients:

Patients who know how to manipulate the system to their advantage, or who are prepared to throw their weight around, can secure preferential treatment. That, said the surgeon, is how the system works: inevitably, it is to some extent responsive to those who exert the greatest pressure on it. Yet it worried him that the consequence might be, as he put it, that the little old lady in social class four will simply say: oh well, that's how things are, I've got to wait. A similar concern about equity was expressed by the public health physician: cases that are given a high profile in the media may lead to the use of costly treatments on unpromising patients while the needs of old people for hip replacements or chiropody go unmet.[41]

Butler does not articulate this in terms of virtues. Had he done so he might have seen that humility – understood as medical professionals not claiming too much and patients not demanding too much – is crucial here. One of the obvious ethical problems of a health service that responds to demand rather than need – after all, demand is much easier to determine and measure than need – is that the most demanding are likely to get a disproportionate amount of available treatment, whereas the least demanding (who may actually be more needy) get the least treatment. As far as the demanding patient may be concerned, selfishness is rewarded. In addition, exaggerated claims about novel treatment made in the media may exacerbate this situation still further. The most demanding patients may also be the ones to search the media – or, more likely, the internet – just in case there are forms of novel (and probably expensive) treatment that they have neglected to demand from their doctors.

In contrast, Daniel Callahan did set his much-criticised proposals in *Setting Limits*, for allocating resources to the elderly, within a context of virtues. Callahan noted at the time that many high-technology, intensive forms of medical treatment were developed in the first instance for young patients who would not otherwise survive, but have gradually (and unsustainably) been offered to the elderly as well. For example, septuagenarians have sometimes been offered kidney transplants (on the grounds that it is wrong to discriminate

---

[41] Butler, *The Ethics of Health Care Rationing*, p. 225.

between potential recipients on the basis of age) even when this meant that younger patients might be denied them. Callahan argued in *Setting Limits* that both elderly patients and the government have duties. On the one hand he proposed that 'the primary aspiration of the aged ... should be to advance not their own welfare but that of the young and the generations to come ... they are stewards of the world they helped fashion in earlier years and must now turn over to others'.[42] On the other, he insisted that 'government has a duty, based on our collective social obligations, to help people live out a natural life span, but not actively to help extend life medically beyond that point ... beyond the point of a natural life span, government should provide only the means necessary for the relief of suffering, not life-extending technology'.[43] Unfortunately his critics tended to note the latter but not the former and accused him at the time of ageism and unfairness to the elderly. In his 'Response to My Critics', Callahan now points out that he did insist earlier that:

The needed changes should be effected, not by compulsion – the young imposing it by force on the unwilling old – but democratically, preceded by a decades-long period of changing our thinking, attitudes and expectations about elderly health care. Those of us still reasonably young should be prepared in the future to impose an age-limit on ourselves.[44]

Of course there are still very real dangers in such proposals. Not least of these is that the severely ill may be induced into feeling guilty for asking too much. The virtue of humility among elderly patients might also be used by an uncaring society as an excuse simply for neglecting them. Yet for Callahan a problem remains:

It is the success of medicine, not its failures, that have created the problem of sustaining and paying for decent health care for the elderly. It is the success of the campaign against ageism, increasing the expectations for everyone for a medically and socially transformed old age, that have added to that problem. If there is any blame to be apportioned it should be directed at our dreams, some of which have come true. It is just that we did not know what that would mean. Now we are finding out.[45]

---

[42] Daniel Callahan, *Setting Limits: Medical Goals in an Aging Society, with 'A Response to my Critics'* (Washington, DC: Georgetown University Press, 1995; first published 1987), p. 82.
[43] Callahan, *Setting Limits*, pp. 137–8. [44] Callahan, *Setting Limits*, p. 227.
[45] Callahan, *Setting Limits*, p. 238.

To return to Butler, he finally does not relate his tentative conclusions about patient needs and demands to his own Christian faith.
Twenty years ago, the theologian Allen Verhey suggested briefly that
both truthfulness and humility are important when allocating scarce
health care resources. Butler did, of course, note in passing the New
Testament's 'dominant moral emphasis on the care of those at the
bottom of the social pile'. For Verhey this meant that 'to provide
ordinary health care to the wealthy because they can pay or to the nice
because we like them or to the promising because of their social
utility while we withhold it from the poor, the outcast, and the
handicapped is not only tragic but unjust'.[46] Recently Lisa Cahill
has also related a biblically generated preferential option for the
marginalised to this debate.[47] Making a second point Verhey argued:

We have been disposed to promise 'everything for everyone' when it comes
to allocation – but our limited resources forbid our fulfilling this promise.
Doctors and nurses may not deny the tragic truth about our world or the
tragic limits of medicine either to their patients or to themselves. The
truthfulness necessary to acknowledge tragedy and the humility necessary
to cope with it can be sustained by piety, for piety knows it is God, not
medicine, who brings in a new age.[48]

Neil Messer has recently used this second point to good effect in
the context of health care rationing, albeit recognising that it certainly does not resolve all of the complex ethical issues involved
here.[49] Verhey, too, has recently insisted that biblical stories (such
as the good Samaritan) cannot 'guarantee unanimity about policy' in
the modern world even among Christians: yet they can motivate and
form 'a prophetic protest against public policies that lead to injustice
in access to health care'.[50]

[46] Allen Verhey, 'Sanctity and Scarcity: the Makings of Tragedy', *The Reformed Journal*, 35
(February 1985), and reprinted in Stephen E. Lammers and Allen Verhey, *On Moral
Medicine: Theological Perspectives in Medical Ethics* (Grand Rapids, MI: William B.
Eerdmans, 1987), p. 655.
[47] Lisa Sowle Cahill, 'Bioethics, Theology, and Social Change', *Journal of Religious Ethics*, 31:3
(2003), p. 377.
[48] Verhey, 'Sanctity and Scarcity', p. 654.
[49] Neil Messer, 'Health Care Resource Allocation and the "Recovery of Virtue"', *Studies in
Christian Ethics*, 18:1 (April 2005).
[50] Allen Verhey, *Remembering Jesus: Christian Community, Scripture and the Moral Life* (Grand
Rapids, MI: William B. Eerdmans, 2002), p. 482.

Returning to the discussion in chapter 1, John Hare's 'moral gap' is also relevant here. It will be recalled that Hare argues that this is the gap that arises from Kant's high moral requirement for individuals combined with his belief that everyone has a propensity not to follow this requirement. In this account, the moral gap is between the requirement that all people should always behave morally in ways that are universalisable and the ubiquitous human propensity to selfishness. Hare identifies several forms that this selfishness takes: self-deception ('I may magnify the intensity of my own preferences, so that they outweigh the preferences of others in the moral calculus'); failures of patience ('I am so convinced of the merit of my cause that I cannot even listen to the claims of another person'); and failures of impartiality ('I do understand the preferences of another, and I do adopt them as hypothetical preferences of my own for the situation in which I would be that person, but I then refuse to give those hypothetical preferences equal weight with my preferences for the actual situation in which I occupy my actual role').[51] Selfishness can take quite subtle forms.

As was seen earlier, Hare also suggests that there are selfish ways to reduce this gap – either by reducing the moral requirement itself (perhaps morality need not be universalisable) or by exaggerating our natural propensities (perhaps humans really are not selfish after all). And it is, doubtless, tempting to use either of these strategies to reduce the ethical dilemmas caused by health care rationing. However, Hare rejects such strategies and argues that his (and Kant's) Christian faith is a more morally appropriate way of addressing this gap. He believes, in contrast to his secular philosophical colleagues, that a notion of God's assistance, or 'divine supplementation', was essential to Kant, and that 'his system does not work unless he is seen as genuinely trying to "make room for faith"'.[52]

This can be illustrated from two other areas of considerable concern to Christian ethics today. The first concerns theories of punishment and prison reform. Anthony Bottoms, like Hare, combines Kantian principles and Christian faith, in his influential ideas about prison

[51] John Hare, *The Moral Gap* (Oxford: Clarendon Paperbacks, Oxford University Press, 1997), p. 25.
[52] Hare, *Moral Gap*, p. 2.

reform. He examines carefully the notion of 'humane containment' developed by Roy King and Rod Morgan which argued that 'imprisonment should only be used as a last resort', that prisoners 'should be subject to only that degree of security necessary to safeguard the public', and that 'as far as the resources allow, and consistent with the constraints of secure custody, the same general standards which govern the life of offenders in the community should be held to apply to offenders in prison'.[53] Bottoms agrees with these principles, but argues that 'there is a clear feeling within the prison system that, while the concept of humane containment is an essential element in running a prison system (and is obviously to be preferred to inhumane containment), the notion of "containment" is insufficient as a goal ... [it is] ontologically insufficient'.[54] For Bottoms respect and care are essential, but so is hope: 'including the fostering of structures and activities within prisons to enable longer-term prisoners to retain a sense of hope; and the provision of appropriate opportunities for all prisoners to better themselves'.[55] In the research of Byron Johnson reviewed in the previous chapter an even stronger claim is made at this point, namely that faith-based interventions in American prisons can be effective in helping 'prisoners to better themselves'. A key point here is that while prison may (or may not) deter potential criminals, only a moral change can eliminate crime. So, faced with the prospect of imprisonment, the clever thief, for example, may simply become more adept at not being detected and the dumb thief may simply learn to enjoy prison, but, until both come to believe that theft is wrong because it harms other people, theft (and other crimes) and imprisonment will remain. Moral faith in universalisability, and with it a move beyond selfishness, does seem to be a minimum requirement here. For Bottoms a preferential option for the marginalised also clearly motivates his work on prison reform.

The second concerns notions of inequality. A system of prioritising that is not simply based upon a patient's social status or ability to

---

[53] Roy King and Rod Morgan, *The Future of the Prison System* (London: Gower, 1980), pp. 34–7.

[54] Anthony Bottoms, 'The Aims of Imprisonment', *Justice, Guilt and Forgiveness in the Penal System* (Edinburgh: The Centre for Theology and Public Issues, New College, Edinburgh University, 1990), p. 9.

[55] Bottoms, 'The Aims of Imprisonment', p. 18.

pay also requires a shared sense of equity and fairness. Douglas Hicks, in his contribution to New Studies in Christian Ethics, namely *Inequality and Christian Ethics*,[56] uses the secular economist Amartya Sen's notion of 'equality of basic capability' – especially Sen's contention that moral perception is inextricably involved in an adequate understanding of equality and inequality in the world. An equality of basic capability, whether applied to the health service or more widely to society at large, involves qualitative issues and not simply a quantitative provision to satisfy basic needs. Hicks argues that, once this is acknowledged, Christian ethics can contribute at three distinctive levels. First, it provides a moral vision and justification for how inequality matters and why public response is needed. Then it can offer moral examples of Christians who have actively striven against inequality. And, thirdly, Christian ethics provides a particularly compelling moral call to action: at best, Christian communities can transform lives and behaviour towards a greater equality of capability. These three distinctively Christian levels are important for addressing the moral gaps noted in chapter 1, but Hicks avoids making strong claims about them – a proper sense of humility is relevant here too. Religious communities can perhaps reduce the moral gap between theoretical and actual moral communities, but their capacity to do so can easily be exaggerated. At best such communities offer a shared understanding of cosmic order that may still resonate with implicit assumptions about equity and fairness in wider society (especially on health care issues). Yet the fact that these assumptions tend to be implicit rather than explicit remains a matter of concern given a human propensity to selfishness.

So far, the suggestion is that Christian ethics might indeed be able to make a significant contribution to the public debate about health care rationing – firstly by fostering an increase of humility and a decrease of selfishness (among both health care professionals and patients), and secondly by motivating and forming 'a prophetic protest against public policies that lead to injustice in access to health care'. Both humility and justice are also essential to my own understanding of health care ethics. But is that all that Christian ethics can

---

[56] Douglas A. Hicks, *Inequality and Christian Ethics* (Cambridge: Cambridge University Press, 2000).

add to health care ethics today in the public forum of a Western, pluralistic society?

Tristram Engelhardt and Mark Cherry's collection *Allocating Scarce Medical Resources: Roman Catholic Perspectives* explores more ambitious options. Engelhardt argues in his introduction that there are some good reasons for believing that theology is relevant to this particular debate:

Because critical care involves choices in the face of finitude, it invites existential questions regarding the meaning of life, the nature of a good death, and the appropriate use of limited resources. For those who know that the prize of human life is immortality, the question arises of how much must be invested in marginally postponing death or of achieving a very small chance for long-term survival, when the real goal is eternal life.[57]

He also argues that a specifically Roman Catholic perspective about dying has obvious relevance here: 'though a nonbeliever might affirm the goodness of a peaceful unforeseen death, Christians have traditionally prayed for an anticipated death ... recognizing that the most significant threat from serious illness is not death but dying without repentance, unreconciled with God'.[58] Subsequent essays in the book also explore other relevant areas of traditional Roman Catholic teaching in health care ethics, such as the doctrines of proportionalism and double effect and the distinction between 'ordinary' and 'extraordinary' means of treatment.

Yet a fundamental difficulty soon emerges in this book for those who are tempted to claim that theology can offer coherent and distinctive ways of resolving the vexed ethical issues of rationing in health care. Even when theologians can agree to use, for example, the doctrines of proportionalism or double effect or the ordinary/extra-ordinary distinction, they find it notoriously difficult to agree about specific applications. Divisions soon emerge at this level among the different contributors to this book. Several contributors also note another problem for specifically Roman Catholic theologians working in modern medicine. A traditional understanding of natural law theology insists that ethical categories and judgements are the

---

[57] Engelhardt and Cherry, *Allocating Scarce Medical Resources*, p. 4.
[58] Engelhardt and Cherry, *Allocating Scarce Medical Resources*, p. 9.

product of (God-given) human reasoning and that Christians and non-Christians alike have access to them (provided that their reasoning is not distorted by sin or error). Given this understanding, it is not obvious why Roman Catholics should believe that they possess a distinctive ethical standpoint in this or in any other area. At most, theology can reinforce what should be obvious from human reasoning alone. As ever, Engelhardt expresses this objection forcefully: 'every time one presses for a specifically Roman Catholic moral theological suggestion regarding the use of critical care resources, one gets what is almost an indignant reply: "Don't you know, we are by faith committed to reason's ability to disclose morality's content."'[59] Moreover, more than one contributor points out that Roman Catholics have been singularly unsuccessful in the Western world in convincing their own members, let alone other Christians or non-Christians, about the rationality of their traditional teaching on contraception or even abortion.

Because the ethical issues raised by intensive care units form a focus for Engelhardt and Cherry's book, the differences between the contributors can be illustrated by looking carefully at their 'Consensus Statement' on 'Determining Appropriate Critical Care'.[60] The working group that produced this statement had little difficulty agreeing that intensive care units are very expensive compared with other kinds of health care and raise acute issues about the fairness of using scarce resources. Instructively, though, they did have more difficulty agreeing 'about the precise authority of the church's teaching office – the magisterium – in interpreting sources' of moral knowledge. They agreed about the finitude of human life, the redemptive value of suffering, the importance of 'proper preparation for death', the direct relevance of the Fifth Commandment to critical care as well as the commandment to love one's neighbour, that people have a natural right to health care, and the need for practical wisdom. However, on the last they noted that 'although there is much dispute among Catholics about the exact workings of practical wisdom, it deals with issues of proportionality and disproportionality of actions

[59] Engelhardt and Cherry, *Allocating Scarce Medical Resources*, p. 14.
[60] Engelhardt and Cherry, *Allocating Scarce Medical Resources*, pp. 35–9. It was originally published in *Christian Bioethics*.

and projects, not in a narrow technical way but against the horizon of a unified Christian life, well lived'. They also agreed on a crucial change that has taken place in intensive care units:

Critical care was developed to monitor patients who were being stabilized after surgery or trauma. As such, critical care is an essential component of modern medicine – a necessary condition for much surgery and a lifesaver for those needing close monitoring. Critical care can be used for other medical purposes. It can, for example, help to extend the life of a person who is dying from cancer or congestive heart failure or provide a carefully monitored environment for PVS patients. But critical care was not designed for such purposes and likely would not exist if they were the only purposes it served. Patient-centered and justice-based considerations converge to suggest that critical care services should be restricted to patients who can get medical benefit from the careful monitoring critical care provides.

Taken in isolation this paragraph appears to be very similar to the conclusions on withholding and withdrawing nutrition and hydration from PVS patients (discussed in chapter 4) of both the 1998 Lambeth Conference of Bishops and the Medical Ethics Committee of the British Medical Association. The former, after all, resolved that 'to withhold or withdraw excessive medical treatment or intervention (e.g. life support) may be appropriate where there is no reasonable prospect of recovery'.[61] And the latter decided that 'if treatment [including artificial nutrition and hydration] fails, or ceases, to give a net benefit to the patient (or if the patient has completely refused the treatment) ... [it] may, ethically and legally, be withheld or withdrawn, and the goal of medicine should shift to the palliation of symptoms'.[62] However, it is not at all clear that the Consensus Statement really does intend this, since a subsequently agreed point is as follows:

Medical treatment, including that which makes use of evidence-based medicine, is distinct from and not as morally basic as basic care. The former can be terminated for patient-based reasons, futility, or justice-based reasons. The latter may never be completely terminated: that would be abandonment of a needy human being.

---

[61] *The Official Report of the Lambeth Conference 1998* (Harrisburg, PA: Morehouse Publishing, 1999), p. 104.

[62] British Medical Association, *Withholding and Withdrawing Life-Prolonging Medical Treatment* (London: BMJ Books, 1999), para 1.

The problem here is to find an agreed way of making this distinction between 'basic care' and 'medical treatment'. Clearly most people would regard surgery, say, as indisputably 'medical treatment' and the provision of food and water as 'basic care'. But what if the latter is delivered through a naso-gastric tube and evacuated using enemas (thus involving medical interventions)? At what stage does 'care' become 'intensive' and thus 'treatment' (and thus something that may be withheld or withdrawn)? Within Catholic theology it is precisely at this point that the doctrines of proportionalism and double effect and the ordinary/extraordinary distinction are deployed. Yet on each of these the various contributors to *Allocating Scarce Medical Resources* show that they have very profound differences. It is with this crucial point of disagreement that the Consensus Statement concludes:

The forty-year-long debates among Roman Catholic moralists focused on proportionalism and double effect are represented among the Catholic moralists in this working group, and have not been settled among us by our discussions about limiting critical care. These disagreements concerning basic moral concepts are likely to mark differences in the interpretation of the Fifth Commandment and of its application in casuistry. Although we did not find important areas of the specific issue of limiting critical care to be affected by these differences, the suspicion remains that there are many particular cases of withholding and limiting treatment where the disagreements on Catholic moral theory would lead to contrary judgments.

Judged from the outside, the only surprise in this conclusion is that the working group 'did not find important areas of the specific issue of limiting critical care to be affected by these differences'. Perhaps this was because they carefully omitted any reference to 'withdrawing' non-benefiting patients from intensive care units. Or perhaps it was because they avoided the issue of the status of artificial nutrition/hydration. Or perhaps, again, it was that they never discussed appropriate penalties for Catholic doctors acting in ways contrary to their 'consensus'. Had they done any of these things they might have discovered some very important differences on limiting critical care.

Once again, one of the most troublesome features of Engelhardt's Christian approach to health care ethics is that it deliberately fuels so-called 'culture wars'. First it pits Christians against the 'secular' world and then it pits Christians against Christians. Perhaps Christians need to learn a little more humility ourselves. It seems to me highly unlikely that Christians will be able convincingly to resolve the difficult and complex ethical issues involved in health care rationing in the West. Nevertheless, we can still make an important contribution to the public debate. Together we might be able to say that humility – understood as medical professionals not claiming too much and patients not demanding too much – is finally essential if we are seriously to engage with health care rationing in Western pluralistic (and deeply privileged) societies.

Conclusion

If health care ethics is to have widespread relevance today in the public forum of a Western, pluralistic society, it manifestly cannot be based solely upon Christian faith. The globalised nature of modern medicine and the multi-cultural composition of health care professionals in Western countries clearly preclude this. For a while the four-principles approach, pioneered successfully in Tom Beauchamp and James Childress' *Principles of Biomedical Ethics*, seemed to offer a 'faith-free' approach to health care ethics that could be relevant and adequate in the public forum. Yet it has been seen that this approach, although still useful, is now widely regarded as too 'thin'. Increasingly it is recognised that virtues are needed alongside principles in an adequate account of health care ethics. And, once this is acknowledged, it becomes more questionable whether health care ethics should remain fastidiously 'faith free'. It is, after all, faith communities around the world that have traditionally played a major role in fostering and embedding virtues. It is even arguable that, despite a number of purely secular attempts, it is faith communities (despite their many frailties) that still have the more enduring record of fostering and embedding virtues.

Be that as it may, if health care ethics is to take adequate account of virtues as well as principles, it may need to pay more attention to those virtues that can be found in a number of faith traditions. Despite the antagonism of theological purists, I have suggested throughout this book that the virtues present in the Synoptic healing stories – compassion, care, faith and humility – can also be found in other theistic traditions and even beyond these traditions. I hope that others, better equipped than myself, will be encouraged to explore this suggestion in depth in their own faith or humanistic tradition.

If it is so, and if these virtues can then be used more explicitly within health care ethics, then I believe that the latter will be deepened and enriched. A combination of the virtues of compassion, care, faith and humility, with the principles of autonomy, justice, non-maleficence and beneficence, provides a much 'thicker' account of health care ethics, with greater critical depth, than either virtues or principles can on their own.

Research within clinical practice might be used to illustrate this claim. Good clinical practice starts with the explicit recognition of compassion, understood as a response to the vulnerable and a determination to help them if at all possible. This determination might also encourage clinicians to do research to help others as well. Clinical practice – and especially clinical research – that lacks compassion soon becomes cold, shallow and 'clinical' in the pejorative sense. Doubtless there are many factors that attract individuals to become clinical researchers, but compassion ought to be (and, fortunately, often is) crucial. It is because of the primacy of compassion that clinicians can often become so tenacious on behalf of their patients and so impatient about wider issues of resource allocation. It is 'their' vulnerable patients who demand their research and clinical attention, so it is difficult to give sufficient consideration to a scarce resource that might need to be allocated fairly to others instead. Compassion also inspires the good clinician to act altruistically and sometimes to override her/his own principled scruples.

Good clinical practice is also concerned to care for and care about patients as persons and not to regard them simply as objects of research. Compassion in clinical practice does need the structures of care to be effective and care needs compassion to direct it aright. Nevertheless, compassion for vulnerable individuals can sometimes be at odds with structures of care designed to bring lasting political or social change. It has been argued that clinical practice in the context of those living with HIV and AIDS must indeed be founded upon compassion. Yet there are socio-political factors involved in the global spread of this virus that should not be ignored even within clinically based research. The clinical researcher working in this context must care compassionately for individual patients, treating them with respect as vulnerable persons. But she/he may still believe that the common good requires determined and possibly unwelcome epidemiological research and action in order to reduce the spread of infection.

Treating patients as persons within clinical research also requires attention to the principles of non-maleficence, beneficence and autonomy. Non-maleficence suggests that a proposed research project involving human participants should not cause them harm. To take an extreme example, research projects seeking to interview child abusers face particularly difficult problems since they may uncover evidence which incriminates those being interviewed, but which serves to protect other people. Such research, although ethically contentious, may still be allowable, but it does need very careful ethical inspection and monitoring. Other research projects might risk physical danger. For example, there has been much discussion in bioscience about the potential risks to people of genetic release, that is about the danger of genetically changed organisms escaping or being released into the body or the environment. At a less dramatic level, questionnaire-surveys may contain unnecessarily intrusive and/or personal questions.

Beneficence suggests that research projects, especially those involving people, should strive positively to bring benefit. Even if no harm is being done, good research should still aim to benefit people or their environment, particularly when it involves the use of other people's time. So research involving human participants which has no clear objectives about benefit, but which is simply undertaken out of curiosity, would be difficult to support if it was in any way intrusive.

Autonomy suggests that, when there are human participants in research projects, they should be treated with respect; they should be properly informed with sufficient and understandable information and space for patients who have the capacity to make a settled choice about medical interventions on themselves, to do so responsibly in a manner considerate to others; they should give their consent voluntarily and without coercion; they should have their confidentiality fully respected; and they should later have the option of feedback about the findings of the research project. In short people should be treated as people and not simply as research objects. Properly informed consent – or, perhaps better, properly informed patient choice – causes many problems in research projects and may require careful mechanisms to ensure that confidentiality for participants is assured. Some projects are so complex that it is difficult to get properly *informed* choice/consent. For example, the genome project is showing just how complicated human genetic inheritance is. Would any programme of widespread genetic screening be able adequately to inform all those taking part? So far this has proved very difficult, given that such information often has little therapeutic relevance at present and yet may damage a patient's prospects of insurance or even employment. In other types of research it may be claimed that it is necessary to withhold some information from those taking part in order to avoid distorting the research itself. Again, what about those with learning disabilities? Many of the most difficult cases involve the study of those with severe learning disabilities. How does one properly gain informed consent from this group of people? Yet, in a society that is increasingly educated, informed choice/ consent and respect for autonomy and confidentiality have become ever more important.

Trust or faith is also crucial to good clinical research at several different levels. At the most basic the patient is expected to trust that the clinician does have her/his well-being at heart. She/he especially needs to be assured that this is so in the context of clinical practice linked directly with research. Clinicians conducting research against the interests of their patients (or acting as agents of totalitarian governments) are now widely vilified in health care ethics. At another level faith involves a mutual relationship or covenant between clin- ician and patient, with the clinician respecting the autonomy and well-being of the patient and the patient that of the clinician. And, at a deeper level still, faith involves the most personal beliefs and commitments of both patient and clinician. It is at this level that faith and well-being may be most intimately related to each other.

Justice suggests that research projects should also take into con- sideration the concerns of the whole of society and should be parti- cularly vigilant about minority groups that might be disadvantaged by the research. The relative distribution of resources for research projects is often contentious for this reason. Should large amounts of money be used for research on genetic disabilities that involve a small number of people, or upon heart disease, which involves many more? Will some research projects benefit people in relatively affluent countries to the disadvantage of those in the poorest countries?

Such questions have sometimes been raised about research projects on genetically improved food resources. Do these resources finally disadvantage the poor and make them ever more dependent upon rich countries' patents, products and even fertilisers? In human genetic research it is also important to be sensitive to the fact that research on people with genetic disorders has implications for their wider families. At a global level, questions of justice also involve environmental questions. For example, genetically improved resources might have an adverse effect upon ecological balances and biodiversity.

Finally this understanding of health care ethics takes the virtue of humility into account. Patients can demand too much and clinical researchers can claim too much: humility is important for both patients and researchers. More than that, clinical researchers may be tempted to claim too much precisely because their patients demand too much. Or, more perniciously, they may be tempted to claim too much in order to encourage their patients to become participants in their research projects. In areas of novel research requiring considerable investment (especially in areas of biotechnology) this temptation can be very real. Yet good clinical practice does finally require a sense of humility, especially in a context of compassionate care.

Compassionate, faithful and humble care – fostered and embedded within moral communities as suggested by the doxological front cover of this book – can deepen and enrich an account of health care ethics instructed by the principles of autonomy, justice, non-maleficence and beneficence. The latter are important. They are principles that properly inform health care ethics today. They have helped to structure moral debate in a pluralistic society and have served to remind those engaged in health care ethics of what is properly required. However, the virtues of compassion, care, faith and humility go further and deeper.

Bibliography of works cited

Allen, Joseph, *Love and Conflict: a Covenantal Model of Christian Ethics*, Nashville: Abingdon Press, 1984

Anglican Communion, *The Official Report of the Lambeth Conference 1998*, Harrisburg, PA: Morehouse Publishing, 1999

Arberry, Arthur J., *The Koran Interpreted*, Oxford: Oxford University Press, 1998

Ashley, Benedict M. and Kevin D. O'Rourke, *Health Care and Ethics: a Theological Analysis*, Washington, DC: Georgetown University Press, 4th edition, 1996

Asser, S. and R. Swan, 'Child Fatalities from Religious-Motivated Medical Neglect', *Pediatrics*, 101, 1998, pp. 625–9

Badham, Paul, 'Should Christians Accept the Validity of Voluntary Euthanasia', in Robin Gill (ed.), *Euthanasia and the Churches*, London: Cassell, 1998, pp. 41–59

Banner, Michael, *Christian Ethics and Contemporary Moral Problems*, Cambridge: Cambridge University Press, 1999

Barrett, C. K., *The Gospel According to St John: an Introduction with Commentary and Notes on the Greek Text*, London: SPCK, 1967

Beauchamp, Tom L. and James F. Childress, *Principles of Biomedical Ethics*, Oxford and New York: Oxford University Press, 4th edition, 1994

Beckford, James A. and Thomas Luckmann (eds.), *The Changing Face of Religion*, London: Sage, 1989

Bennett, Rebecca, Heather Draper and Lucy Firth, 'Ignorance is Bliss? HIV and Moral Duties and Legal Duties to Forewarn', *Journal of Medical Ethics*, 26:1, 2000, pp. 9–15

Borg, Marcus J., *Conflict, Holiness and Politics in the Teaching of Jesus*, Harrisburg, PA: Trinity Press International, 2nd edition, 1998

Bottoms, Anthony, 'The Aims of Imprisonment', *Justice, Guilt and Forgiveness in the Penal System*, Edinburgh: The Centre for Theology and Public Issues, New College, Edinburgh University, 1990

British Medical Association, *Our Genetic Future: the Science and Ethics of Genetic Technology*, Oxford: Oxford University Press, 1992
  Withholding and Withdrawing Life-Prolonging Medical Treatment, London: BMJ Books, 1999 (updated 2001)
  'Public Debate about Euthanasia', 3 December 2003: http://www.bma. org.uk/ap.nsf/Content/MedicalEthicsTomorrowConfpapers
  Medical Ethics Today, London: BMJ Books, 2004
Brown, Colin, *Miracles and the Critical Mind*, Grand Rapids, MI: William B. Eerdmans, 1984
  That You May Believe: Miracles and Faith Then and Now, Grand Rapids, MI: William B. Eerdmans, 1985
Browning, Don, Bonnie Miller-McLemore, Pamela Couture, Bernie Lyon and Robert Franklin, *From Culture Wars to Common Ground*, Louisville, KY: Westminster/John Knox, 1997
Bruce, Steve (ed.), *Religion and Modernization*, Oxford: Oxford University Press, 1992
Burke, Derek, 'Genetic Engineering of Food', in Fraser Watts (ed.), *Christians and Bioethics*, London: SPCK, 2000, pp. 21–34
Butler, John, *The Ethics of Health Care Rationing: Principles and Practices*, London: Cassell, 1999
Byrd, R. C., 'Positive Therapeutic Effects of Intercessory Prayer in a Coronary Care Unit Population', *Southern Medical Journal*, 81, 1988, pp. 826–9
Cahill, Lisa Sowle, 'Bioethics, Theology, and Social Change', *Journal of Religious Ethics*, 31:3, 2003, pp. 363–98
  'Biotech Justice: Catching up with the Real World Order', *Hastings Center Report*, 33:5, 2003, pp. 34–44
Callahan, Daniel, *Setting Limits: Medical Goals in an Aging Society, with 'A Response to my Critics'*, Washington, DC: Georgetown University Press, 1995 (first published 1987)
  'Principlism and Communitarianism', *Journal of Medical Ethics*, 29:5, 2003, pp. 287–91
Campbell, Alastair V., 'Response', in Robin Gill (ed.), *Euthanasia and the Churches*, London: Cassell, 1998, pp. 113–16
  'The Virtues (and Vices) of the Four Principles', *Journal of Medical Ethics*, 29:5, 2003, pp. 292–6
Carrette, Jeremy and Philip King, *Selling Spirituality?*, London: Routledge, 2005
Casanova, José, 'Beyond European and American Exceptionalisms', in Grace Davie, Paul Heelas and Linda Woodhead (eds.), *Predicting Religion: Christian, Secular and Alternative Futures*: Aldershot, Hants: Ashgate, 2003, pp. 17–29

Cavanaugh, Thomas, 'Double Effect and the Ethical Significance of Distinct Volitional States', *Christian Bioethics*, 3:2, 1997, pp. 131–41

Chalmers, J., 'The Criminalisation of HIV Transmission', *Journal of Medical Ethics*, 28:3, 2002, pp. 160–3

Chapman, Audrey R., *Unprecedented Choices: Religious Ethics at the Frontiers of Genetic Science*, Minneapolis: Fortress Press, 1999

Clark, Stephen R. L., *Biology and Christian Ethics*, Cambridge: Cambridge University Press, 2000

Cook, Christopher C. H., *Alcohol, Addiction and Christian Ethics*, Cambridge: Cambridge University Press, 2006

Cragg, Kenneth, *The Mind of the Qu'ran*, London: Allen & Unwin, 1973

Crocket, Alasdair and Richard O'Leary (eds.), *Patterns and Processes of Religious Change in Modern Industrial Societies – Europe and the United States*, Lampeter: Mellen, 2004

Cronin, Kieran, *Rights and Christian Ethics*, Cambridge: Cambridge University Press, 1992

Davies, Oliver, *A Theology of Compassion*, London: SCM Press, 2001

Davies, W. D. and Dale C. Allison Jr, *A Critical Commentary on the Gospel According to Saint Matthew*, vol. II, Edinburgh: T. & T. Clark, 1991

Deane-Drumond, Celia, *Genetics and Christian Ethics*, Cambridge: Cambridge University Press, 2005

Doyal, Len, 'The Role of the Public in Health Care Rationing', *Critical Public Health*, 4, 1993, pp. 49–52

'Needs, Rights and Equity: Moral Quality in Healthcare Rationing', *Quality in Health Care*, 4, 1995, pp. 273–83

Dube, Musa W. (ed.), *HIV/AIDS and the Curriculum: Methods of Integrating HIV/AIDS in Theological Programmes*, Geneva: World Council of Churches Publications, 2003

Dunn, James D. G., 'Jesus and Purity: an Ongoing Debate', *New Testament Studies*, 48, 2002, pp. 449–67

Dunstan, G. R. review of *On Moral Medicine* in *Journal of Medical Ethics*, 26:2, 2000, p. 77

Durkheim, Emile, *The Elementary Forms of the Religious Life* [1915], London: George Allen and Unwin, 1976

Dworkin, Ronald, *Life's Dominion: an Argument about Abortion and Euthanasia*, London: Harper Collins, 1993

ECUSA, *Assisted Suicide and Euthanasia: the Washington Report*, Harrisburg, PA: Morehouse Publishing, 1997

Engelhardt, Jr, H. Tristram, 'Towards a Christian Bioethics', *Christian Bioethics*, 1:1, 1995, pp. 1–10

The Foundations of Bioethics, New York: Oxford University Press, 2nd edition, 1996

'The Dechristianization of Christian Hospital Chaplaincy: Some Bioethics Reflections on Professionalization, Ecumenization, and Secularization', *Christian Bioethics*, 9:1, 2003, pp. 139–59

Engelhardt, Jr, H. Tristram and Mark J. Cherry (eds.), *Allocating Scarce Medical Resources: Roman Catholic Perspectives*, Washington, DC: Georgetown University Press, 2002

Evans, C. F., *Saint Luke*, London and Philadelphia: SCM Press and Trinity Press, 1990

Evans, John H., *Play God? Human Genetic Engineering and the Rationalization of Public Bioethical Debate*, Chicago: Chicago University Press, 2002

Farley, Margaret A., *Compassionate Respect: a Feminist Approach to Medical Ethics and Other Questions*, New York and Mahwah, NJ: Paulist Press, 2002

Fergusson, David, *Community, Liberalism and Christian Ethics*, Cambridge: Cambridge University Press, 1998

Fletcher, Joseph, *Situation Ethics*, Philadelphia and London: Westminster and SCM Press, 1966

Frankena, W. K., 'The Potential of Theology for Ethics', in E. E. Shelp (ed.), *Theology and Bioethics*, Dordrecht: D. Reidel, 1985, pp. 49–64

Fulford, K. W. M., 'No More Medical Ethics', in K. W. M. Fulford, Grant R. Gillett and Janet Martin Soskice (eds.), *Medicine and Moral Reasoning*, Cambridge: Cambridge University Press, 1994, pp. 193–205

Gascoigne, Robert, *The Public Forum and Christian Ethics*, Cambridge: Cambridge University Press, 2001

Gilkey, Langdon, *On Niebuhr: a Theological Study*, Chicago: University of Chicago Press, 2001

Gill, Robin, *Competing Convictions*, London: SCM Press, 1989

Moral Leadership in a Postmodern Age, Edinburgh: T. & T. Clark, 1997

'Euthanasia – Response to Paul Badham', *Studies in Christian Ethics*, 11:1, Edinburgh: T. & T. Clark, 1998, pp. 19–23

Churchgoing and Christian Ethics, Cambridge: Cambridge University Press, 1999

The 'Empty' Church Revisited, Aldershot, Hants: Ashgate, 2003

Gillon, Raanan (ed.), *Principles of Health Care Ethics*, London: Wiley, 1985

Gillon, Raanan, 'Ethics Needs Principles – Four Can Encompass the Rest – and Respect for Autonomy Should be "First Among Equals"', *Journal of Medical Ethics*, 29:5, 2003, pp. 307–12

Glover, Jonathan, *Humanity: a Moral History of the Twentieth Century*, London: Jonathan Cape, 1999

Graham, Gordon, *Evil and Christian Ethics*. Cambridge: Cambridge University Press, 2001

Hallett, Garth, *Priorities and Christian Ethics*, Cambridge: Cambridge University Press, 1998

Halmos, Paul, *The Faith of the Counsellors*, London: Constable, 1965

Hammond, Philip E. (ed.), *The Sacred in a Secular Age*, Berkeley: University of California Press, 1984

Hare, John, *The Moral Gap*, Oxford: Clarendon Paperbacks, Oxford University Press, 1997

Harris, John, 'Consent and End of Life Decisions', *Journal of Medical Ethics*, 29:1, 2003, pp. 10–15

Harvey, Peter, *An Introduction to Buddhism*, Cambridge: Cambridge University Press, 1990

Hauerwas, Stanley, *A Community of Character: Toward a Constructive Christian Social Ethic*, Notre Dame, IN: University of Notre Dame Press, 1981

    Suffering Presence, Notre Dame, IN, and Edinburgh: University of Notre Dame Press, 1986 and T. & T. Clark, 1988

    Naming the Silences, Grand Rapids, MI: William B. Eerdmans, 1990

    With the Grain of the Universe: the Church's Witness and Natural Theology, Grand Rapids, MI: Brazos Press, 2001

Hicks, Douglas A., *Inequality and Christian Ethics*, Cambridge: Cambridge University Press, 2000

Hinnells, John R. and Roy Porter (eds.), *Religion, Health and Suffering*, London and New York: Kegan Paul International, 1999

Hollenbach, David, *The Common Good and Christian Ethics*, Cambridge: Cambridge University Press, 2002

Hooker, Morna D., *The Gospel According to St Mark*, London: A. & C. Black, 1991

Horton, John and Susan Mendus (eds.), *After MacIntyre: Critical Perspectives on the Work of Alasdair MacIntyre*, Oxford and Notre Dame, IN: Polity Press and University of Notre Dame Press, 1994

Howe, Kenneth, *Religion, Spirituality and Older People*, Centre for Policy on Ageing, 25–31 Ironmonger Row, London, ECIV 3QP, 1999

Hummer, Robert A., Richard G. Rogers, Charles B. Nam and Christopher G. Ellison, 'Religious Involvement and US Adult Mortality', *Demography*, 36:2, 1999, pp. 273–85

Jeremias, J., *The Parables of Jesus*, London: SCM Press, 1963

Johnson, Byron R., Ralph Brett Tompkins and Derek Webb, *Objective Hope: Assessing the Effectiveness of Faith-Based Organizations: a Review of the Literature*, Philadelphia: Center for Research on Religion and Urban Civil Society, University of Pennsylvania, 2001 [www.crrucs.org]

Jones, David Albert, *The Soul of the Embryo: an Enquiry into the Status of the Human Embryo in the Christian Tradition*, London: Continuum, 2004

Juergensmeyer, Mark, *Terror in the Mind of God: the Global Rise of Violence*, Berkeley: University of California Press, 3rd edition, 2003

Kee, Howard Clark, *Miracle in the Early Christian World*, New Haven, CT: Yale University Press, 1983

  Medicine, Miracle and Magic in New Testament Times, Cambridge: Cambridge University Press, 1986

Kimmelman, Jonathan, 'Recent Developments in Gene Transfer: Risk and Ethics', *British Medical Journal*, 330:53, 8 January 2005, pp. 79–82

King, Roy and Rod Morgan, *The Future of the Prison System*, London: Gower, 1980

Kleinman, Arthur, *Patients and Healers in the Context of Culture*, Berkeley: University of California Press, 1980

Koenig, Harold G., *Spirituality in Patient Care*, Philadelphia and London: Templeton Foundation Press, 2002

Koenig, Harold G., Judith C. Hayes, David B. Larson, Linda K. George, Harvey Jay Cohen, Michael E. McCullough, Keith G. Meador and Dan G. Blazer, 'Does Religious Attendance Prolong Survival? A Six-Year Follow-up Study of 3,968 Older Adults', *Journal of Gerontology: Medical Sciences*, 54A:7, 1999, M370–M376

Koenig, Harold G., Michael E. McCullough and David B. Larson, *Handbook of Religion and Health*, New York: Oxford University Press, 2001

Krause, Neale and Keith M. Wulff, 'Religious Doubt and Health: Exploring the Potential Dark Side of Religion', *Sociology of Religion*, 65:1, 2004, pp. 35–56

Kulczycki, Andrzej, *The Abortion Debate in the World Arena*, London: Macmillan, 1999

Küng, Hans and Walter Jens, *A Dignified Dying*, London: SCM Press, 1995

Lammers, Stephen E., 'On Stanley Hauerwas: Theology, Medical Ethics, and the Church', in Allen Verhey and Stephen E. Lammers (eds.), *Theological Voices in Medical Ethics*, Grand Rapids, MI: William B. Eerdmans, 1993, pp. 74–6

Lee, Simon, *Uneasy Ethics*, London: Pimlico, 2003

Lott, Eric, *Healing Wings: Acts of Jesus for Human Wholeness*, Bangalore, India: Asian Trading Corporation, 1998

Lovin, Robin W., *Reinhold Niebuhr and Christian Realism*, Cambridge and New York: Cambridge University Press, 1995

  'Reinhold Niebuhr in Contemporary Scholarship: A Review Essay', *Journal of Religious Ethics*, 31:3, 2003, pp. 489–505

M'Neile, A. H., *The Gospel According to St Matthew*, London and New York: Macmillan and St Martin's Press, 1965

MacIntyre, Alasdair, *After Virtue: a Study in Moral Theory*, London: Duckworth, 2nd edition, 1985

'A Partial Response to my Critics', in John Horton and Susan Mendus (eds.), *After MacIntyre: Critical Perspectives on the Work of Alasdair MacIntyre*, Oxford and Notre Dame, IN: Polity Press and University of Notre Dame Press, 1994, pp. 283–304

Maguire, Daniel C., *Sacred Choices: the Right to Contraception and Abortion in Ten World Religions*, Minneapolis: Fortress Press, 2001

Malina, Bruce J., *The New Testament World*, Louisville, KY: Westminster John Knox, 3rd edition, 2001

Marshall, Christopher D., *Faith as a Theme in Mark's Narrative*, Cambridge: Cambridge University Press, 1989

Marshall, I. Howard, *The Gospel of Luke*, Exeter: Paternoster, 1978

May, William F., 'Code, Covenant, Contract or Philanthropy: a Basis for Professional Ethics', *Hastings Center Report*, December 1975

The Physician's Covenant: Images of the Healer in Medical Ethics, Philadelphia: Westminster Press, 1983

Meilaender, Gilbert, 'On William May: Corrected Vision for Medical Ethics', in Allen Verhey and Stephen E. Lammers (eds.), *Theological Voices in Medical Ethics*, Grand Rapids, MI: William B. Eerdmans, 1993, pp. 114–19

Body, Soul and Bioethics, Notre Dame, IN: University of Notre Dame Press, 1995

Bioethics: a Primer for Christians, Grand Rapids, MI: William B. Eerdmans, 1996

Melinsky, M. A. H., *Healing Miracles: an Examination from History and Experience of the Place of Miracle in Christian Thought and Medical Practice*, London: Mowbray, 1968

Messer, Neil (ed.), *Theological Issues in Bioethics*, London: DLT, 2002

Messer, Neil, 'Health Care Resource Allocation and the "Recovery of Virtue"', *Studies in Christian Ethics*, 18:1, April 2005

Milbank, John, *Theology and Social Theory*, Oxford: Blackwell, 1990

Mills John Orme Introduction to the reprinted David Martin, John Orme Mills and W. S. F. Pickering (eds.), *Sociology and Theology: Alliance and Conflict*, Leiden and Boston: Brill, 2004

Nichols, Aidan, 'Non Tali Auxilio: John Milbank's Suasion to Orthodoxy', *New Blackfriars*, 73:861, June 1992, pp. 326–32

Norman, Richard, 'Applied Ethics: What is Applied to What?', *Utilitas*, 12:2, 2000, pp. 119–36

Numbers, Ronald L. and Darrel W. Amundsen (eds.), *Caring and Curing: Health and Medicine in the Western Religious Traditions*, London and New York: Macmillan, 1986

O'Neill, Onora, *Autonomy and Trust in Bioethics*, Cambridge: Cambridge University Press, 2002

A Question of Trust, Reith Lectures 2002: www.bbc.co.uk/radio4/reith2002

'Some Limits of Informed Consent', *Journal of Medical Ethics*, 29:1, 2003, pp. 4–7

Osborn, Lawrence and Andrew Walker (eds.), *Harmful Religion: an Exploration of Religious Abuse*, London: SPCK 1997

Pattison, E. Mansell, 'Systems Pastoral Care', *Journal of Pastoral Care*, 26:1, 1972, pp. 3–14

Pellegrino, Edmund D. and Alan I. Faden (eds.), *Jewish and Catholic Bioethics: an Ecumenical Dialogue*, Washington, DC: Georgetown University Press, 1999

Pilch, John, 'Understanding Healing in the Social World of Early Christianity', *Biblical Theology Bulletin*, 22:1, 1992, pp. 26–33
Healing in the New Testament: Insights from Medical and Mediterranean Anthropology, Minneapolis: Fortress Press, 2000

Pinching, Anthony J., 'Commentary: the Ethics of Anonymised HIV Testing of Pregnant Women: A Reappraisal', *Journal of Medical Ethics*, 26:1, 2000, pp. 22–4

Pinching, Anthony J., Roger Higgs and Kenneth M. Boyd, 'The Impact of AIDS on Medical Ethics', *Journal of Medical Ethics*, 26:1, 2000, pp. 3–8

Plant, Raymond, 'Foreword', in William F. Storrar and Andrew R. Morton (eds.), *Public Theology for the 21st Century*, Edinburgh: T. & T. Clark, 2004, pp. x–xi

Pope, Stephen J., 'Natural Law and Christian Ethics', in Robin Gill (ed.), *The Cambridge Companion to Christian Ethics*, Cambridge: Cambridge University Press, 2001

Porter, Jean, *Moral Action and Christian Ethics*, Cambridge: Cambridge University Press, 1995

Power, Michael, *The Audit Society*, Oxford: Oxford University Press, 1996

Rae, Scott B. and Paul M. Cox (eds.), *Bioethics: a Christian Approach in a Pluralistic Age*, Grand Rapids, MI: William B. Eerdmans, 1999

Risen, James and Judy L. Thomas, *Wrath of Angels: the American Abortion War*, New York: Basic Books, Perseus Book Group, 1999

Robbins, Vernon, *The Tapestry of Early Christian Discourse: Rhetoric, Society and Ideology*, London: Routledge, 1996

Robinson, J. M., *The Problem of History in Mark*, London: SCM Press, 1957

Sandeen, E., *The Roots of Fundamentalism: British and American Millenarianism, 1800–1930*, Chicago: University of Chicago Press, 1970

Schaefer, Nancy A., 'Making the Rulers Tremble!: Morris Cerullo World Evangelism's 1994 Mission to London Revival', in Marion Bowman (ed.), *Healing and Religion*, Enfield Lock, Middlesex: Hisarlik Press, 2000, pp. 23–34

Schweiker, William, *Responsibility and Christian Ethics*, Cambridge: Cambridge University Press, 1995
  Theological Ethics and Global Dynamics: In the Time of Many Worlds, New York and London: Blackwell, 2004
Short, R. V., 'Male Circumcision: a Scientific Perspective: the Health Benefits of Male Circumcision are Wide Ranging', *Journal of Medical Ethics*, 30:3, 2004, p. 241
Sloan, R. P., E. Bagiella and T. Powell, 'Viewpoint: Religion, Spirituality and Medicine', *The Lancet*, 353, 20 February 1999, pp. 664–7
Smith, David H., 'Professional Commitment to Personal Care: Nurses' Commitments in Care for the Dying', in David H. Smith (ed.), *Caring Well: Religion, Narrative, and Health Care Ethics*, Louisville, KY: Westminster John Knox Press, 2000, pp. 221–38
Spriggs, M. and T. Charles, 'Should HIV Discordant Couples Have Access to Assisted Reproductive Technologies?', *Journal of Medical Ethics*, 29:6, 2000, pp. 325–9
Stirrat, Gordon M. and Robin Gill, 'Autonomy in Medical Ethics After O'Neill', *Journal of Medical Ethics*, 31:2, 2005, pp. 127–30
Taylor, Charles, *Sources of the Self: the Making of the Modern Identity*, Cambridge, MA: Harvard University Press, 1989
  'Justics After Virtue', in John Horton and Susan Mendus (eds.), *After MacIntyre: Critical Perspectives on the Work of Alasdair MacIntyre*, Oxford and Notre Dame, IN: Polity Press and University of Notre Dame Press, 1994, pp. 16–43
Taylor, Vincent, *The Gospel According to St Mark*, London: Macmillan, 1959
Theissen, Gerd, *The Miracle Stories of the Early Christian Tradition*, Edinburgh and Philadelphia: T. & T. Clark and Fortress Press, 1983 (German original 1974)
Toulmin, Stephen, 'The Tyranny of Principles: Regaining the Ethics of Discretion', *Hastings Center Report*, December 1981
UNAIDS, *A Report of a Theological Workshop Focusing on HIV- and AIDS-related Stigma*, Geneva: UNAIDS, 2005: http://www.unaids.org
Verhey, Allen, 'Sanctity and Scarcity: the Makings of Tragedy', *The Reformed Journal*, 35, February 1985, and reprinted in Stephen E. Lammers and Allen Verhey, *On Moral Medicine: Theological Perspectives in Medical Ethics*, Grand Rapids, MI: William B. Eerdmans, 1987, pp. 653–7
  Remembering Jesus: Christian Community, Scripture and the Moral Life, Grand Rapids, MI: William B. Eerdmans, 2002
WCC, *Facing AIDS: the Challenge, the Churches' Response*, Geneva: World Council of Churches Publications, 1997
Weaver, Darlene Fozard, *Self Love and Christian Ethics*, Cambridge: Cambridge University Press, 2002

Williams, Preston N., 'Christian Realism and the Ephesian Suggestion', *Journal of Religious Ethics*, 25:2, 1997, pp. 233–40

Wokler, Robert, 'Projecting the Enlightenment', in John Horton and Susan Mendus (eds.), *After MacIntyre: Critical Perspectives on the Work of Alasdair MacIntyre*, Oxford and Notre Dame, IN: Polity Press and University of Notre Dame Press, 1994, pp. 108–26

Yao, Xinzhong, *An Introduction to Confucianism*, Cambridge: Cambridge University Press, 2000

Zulueta, Paquita de, 'The Ethics of Anonymised HIV Testing of Pregnant Women: a Reappraisal', *Journal of Medical Ethics*, 26:1, 2000, pp. 16–21

Index

225